KING GLAND PROSTATE

KNOW, CARE & CURE

includes

Homeopathy, Ayurveda, Yoga, Naturopathy, Diet, Acupressure, Magnetotherapy

DR. SHIV DUA

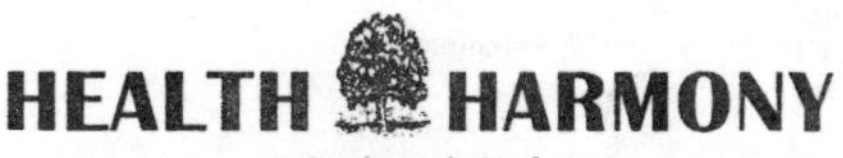

HEALTH HARMONY

An imprint of

B. Jain Publishers (P) Ltd.

USA – Europe – India

KING GLAND PROSTATE — KNOW, CARE AND CURE

First Edition: 2006
4th Impression: 2017

NOTE FROM THE PUBLISHERS
Any information given in this book is not intended to be taken as a replacement for medical advice. Any person requiring medical attention should consult a qualified practitioner or a therapeutist.

Published by Kuldeep Jain for

An imprint of
B. JAIN PUBLISHERS (P) LTD.
D-157, Sector-63, NOIDA-201307, U.P. (INDIA)
Tel.: +91-120-4933333 • *Email:* info@bjain.com
Website: **www.bjain.com**
Registered office: 1921/10, Chuna Mandi, Paharganj, New Delhi-110 055 (India)

Printed in India by
J.J. Offset Printers

ISBN: 978-81-319-0345-2

Dedication

This book is dedicated to my respected father Late Shri Hira Nand Dua who gave me my first lessons in homeopathy. It was he who guided me about the working of the prostate gland. He always called prostate as the 'king' gland of the body.

The book is also dedicated to all "gray haired golden people" who are nearing retirement or leading a retired life.

THANKS

My wife Uma Dua, son Dharmesh, daughter Nilima; Amit, Anuradha, Tanya, Akshay and Aryan for their contribution to enable me to write this book.

Dr. Sanjeev Kumar, B. Sc., BHMS (Gold Medallist). His knowledge on anatomical and physiological aspects of the body always helps and guides me in writing my books.

Dr. R.S. Chandna, Ex-President, H.M.A.I., Faridabad for his cooperation.

All doctors of HMAI, Aligarh unit, namely Drs. B.N. Paul, Anwer Salam, Yogesh Gupta, R. Saraswat, S.K. Gaur, Manish Jain, D.C. Banerjee, R.K. Vashishta, M.C. Banerjee, Niranjan Lal, P.K. Sharma, Sagheer Ahmed, Ashok Vashistha, Rajat Saxena, R.K. Saxena, P.K. Dasgupta, Ravi Sharma, Sunil Gupta and Mrs. Poonam Batra. They conferred continuous confidence in me and invited me to their scientific meets and seminars to impart and exchange views on homeopathy.

Dr. Shiv Dua

M.A., D.I.Hom., HMD (London)

INTRODUCTION

"Prostate is a King gland because queens do not have it. It is a proprietary providence of male's prowess to be called a **'Purash'**. That is why it is called **'PORUSH OR PURASTH Granthi'** in Hindi. Prostate is a symbolic pride depicting youth. When youth is gone, prostate also gets old, wrinkled, enlarged and even diseased."

This is what my father late Shri Hira Nand Dua told me about the prostate gland. He was a true devotee of Homeopathy. A doctor Milava Ram of Dera Ismail Khan, NWFP, Pakistan introduced him to homeopathy and biochemistry. He had some 'Urdu' books published by J.S. Sant Singh of Lahore. After the partition of India when our family shifted to Amritsar, I saw three books with him—Organon, Materia Medica of Kent and Boericke. I do not know how many books he was having while in Pakistan. An Urdu book 'Kamil Sanyasi' (still with me) containing pen-sketches of body's organs was his pride possession. It was this 'Unani' literature that gave me first information about the prostate gland.

In 1995, I wrote an article in Hindi, **"Jab Prostate Granthi Barh Jaye"** and it was published in 'Rajasthan Patrika' (13.10.95); a leading Hindi daily of Rajasthan. Those days I was working in Geological Survey of India and posted in camp Sawar of Dist. Ajmer, Rajasthan. In the evening attended to patients at Bus Stand, Sawar. A small hardware store owner had provided verandah of his shop with table, bench, chair and wooden box to keep my medicines that were distributed free of cost to the people. After this article was published in newspaper, many aged patients having prostate complaints started coming. Before reading this article, they never thought of the existence of this gland and they always held kidneys responsible for their urine problems. The fact is that more than seventy five percent of our male population lives in rural areas and most of them do not know about the names of glands like Prostate. This is unfortunate that people are trained to earn livelihood, trained to keep good health, trained to keep off vices but not trained to know their body parts. Parents tell their children to take milk, butter, ghee or non-vegetarian meals and also about exercise but no one tells them about working of our body. Imparting this knowledge is left to the school teachers. If a student learns something about human body during his study course, prostate does not come up in the primary functioning of body until there is a higher study of medicine.

Even if people are told about the prostate and its connection with sexual activity, they would resort to celibacy or avoid sex rather than going in for treatment or operation. For them, anything connected with urine problems is due to less intake of water or 'Lassi' or 'Chhachh'. In big cities and towns where people are better educated, they are aware of prostate problems but still they avoid its operation, thinking that it is a symbol of their existing sexual power, which they do not want to part with.

In the name of psycho-analysis (propagated by Freud), many doctors say that sexual activity entertains mind and dissolves tensions. It is a materialistic view of modern era and has no scientific basis. Freud does not say that one should indulge in sex only to entertain or erase tensions. His saying is that it should not be suppressed. Indian people are traditionally bound to think that conservation of semen through celibacy means prolonged life and youthfulness.

According to 'Vedas', **loss of semen is death and its absorption in the body is life.** We have two types of secretions - internal and external. Some internal secretions, when absorbed in the body, keep the body healthy and prolong longevity. Man can overcome old age diseases (prostate enlargement or prostate cancer included) by preservation of semen. By its loss, the life is shortened. When an old man, of say seventy years, indulges in prolonged sexual act, his blood pressure increases and when it is difficult to cope up with this increased pressure, it ends in paralysis or brain hemorrhage. This also means that an old man indulging in sex is putting undue pressure on his prostate for release of fluid. Where is the necessity to do so when the efficiency of prostate is on the decline? It is supposed to be left idle. Many doctors do not agree to this argument and say that prostate must be kept active for prolonged life of the gland.

According to ancient Vedic system, the life of man is hundred years. At the age of fifty, he enters *'Vaanprastha ashram.'* After the age of fifty, no one should enter into sexual acts, if he desires to live upto one hundred years. We are Indians and should believe in Indian system of living. Why should we leave our thinking and way of life and adopt western materialism, thinking, eating habits and their sex 'adventures' like anal/oral/unnatural sex? **'We should preserve precious semen after the age of fifty and let it get absorbed in the body to avoid diseases of 'Porush granthi', says the golden Indian philosophy.**

Prostate is an organ that is **most susceptible to cancer** and no one knows when it develops and when to start preventive treatment. No other human organ in our body is so much prone to cancer as is the prostate. In America, more than two lakh men fall victim to prostate cancer each year.

About forty thousand men die of prostate cancer each year in America. When, in a country like America, with advanced medical awareness among people has such a toll of deaths, one can imagine the state of prostate cancer in India. How many Indian men die of prostate cancer? There is no record about it because of lack of data and information fed to the government hospitals. The facilities of curing prostate cancer or removal of gland in the villages and small towns are missing and hence villagers die of cancer without any record of it in dispensaries. Even if the facilities are made available one cannot educate the people on this aspect overnight. In western countries, medical awareness is far superior to eastern countries. USA has government and non-government organizations, which keep record, advise and console patients of cancer, thyroid and prostate etc. They have made societies like Thyroid, Cancer or Prostate Care.

There is a practical problem in diagnosing prostate enlargement and cancer of prostate gland. By the time, the symptoms appear, the gland is already enlarged or having carcinoma. The conventional check systems, pathological tests and electronic gadgets do help but there is still scope for such an investigating tool that could serve the purpose of early diagnosis of this disease. Recently it has been reported that a rapid check system has been installed in Mumbai's Jaslok Hospital that does the JOB!, scanning in seconds. This is done by light speed Volume Computed Tomography called **VCT**, which is the fastest quick-fix diagnostic tool. It enables the doctors to capture the images of the heart and coronary arteries in just five heartbeats. The machine has the potential to change the way diseases are diagnosed and treated. It scans the kidneys in just one second and can perform a complete body scan in ten seconds. At present angiography takes around thirty minutes, brain scan forty five minutes and complete body scan takes two hours.

We are in a world of continuous change in scientific and technical studies. Hopefully, the day is not far when diagnosis of cancer would be made in its budding stage for treatment.

Government has recognized six systems of medicines namely Allopathic, Homeopathic, Ayurvedic, Unani, Sidha and Yoga/Naturopathy. **In this book, Prostate, has been dealt with Homeopathy, Ayurveda and Yoga/Naturopathy so that the readers have options to resort to.** The aim is to bring home cure before surgery is done. If early home treatment is undertaken at the onset of primary symptoms, there is every scope that operation to remove prostate gland is averted.

This book about prostate gland is written to serve those gentlemen who consult doctors for treatment of urine problems and are diagnosed with problems in prostate. Doctors have no time to tell the patients about functioning of the prostate. Even if the problem is explained, patients do not get a correct idea about its care and management. With little knowledge that the problem is with his sexual sphere, he is worried and ashamed of telling his relatives and friends. This book tells about the prostate gland in simple and non-medical language, so that there is no confusion.

The size of the book has been kept small so that one can read it in a single sitting. The utility of the book is for **'old-gold-aged'** patients suffering from prostate diseases and for students or practicing medical professionals. There are ten sections in the book so that one can have complete knowledge of the gland, its diseases and care, management in a quick glance.

25th June 06
2617, Sector-16,
Faridabad-121002

Dr. Shiv Dua
Regd. 4084-B (Haryana),
Phone: 2281764, 09312302205 (M)
E-mail: shiv_duadr@yahoo.co.in

HELLO, I AM YOUR GENTLE, GENTEEL AND GENETIC KING ORGAN, PROSTATE

Sir,

I am your prostate, living in your body in a generative zone. I am situated in the cavity of the true pelvis under the fundus of the bladder and have a base and an apex. If you are fifty years old, I am too fifty years old. My shape is like an English walnut lying in a inverted triangle and weighing about 20 grams (adult). It is variable from 20 to 30 gms. I am almost wrapped around your urethra like a ring fits the finger. Human race is due to my presence in your body. I am also called 'Porush Granthi or Purasth Granthi' in Hindi. I get activated when you do intercourse with your partner. Your testes then produce about 200 million sperms cells and my job is to dilute them with a fluid. This special fluid has enzymes, proteins, sugar and fat to nourish the fragile sperms. It provides alkalinity to overpower the acidic female tract and in this fluid, the sperms can swim towards the female egg. I do not know how I ejaculate my fluid but I definitely get directives from the lower end of your spinal cord. Many more jobs are accomplished on such directives. The sphincter valve of the bladder that opens in the urethra gets closed. My whole body contracts and the two seminal vesicles also get squeezed. The vesicles send about twenty percent of my fluid and the rest less than a teaspoonful goes out through the urethra. I have three lobes lying side-by-side and encased in a capsule. The small urinary tube which empties the bladder crosses through the middle lobe. Any inflammation, hypertrophy and infection or cancer etc. occurring here naturally enlarges these lobes and obstructs the urine flow. When urine is not passing freely, I am very much disturbed because some urine is blocked in the bladder and becomes stagnant. Bacteria grows there and brings many more complications. I cannot tell more about that because my vision is limited to my activities.

When you were thirteen years old, my size was that of an almond weighing about 8 grams. With increase of your age and induction of hormonal signals, my size also got enlarged. At puberty, my weight became doubled. My grapelike clusters of glands began making seminal fluid for storing in my muscled pouch. I am of normal size by the age of twenty years. At the age of fifty, I am twenty percent more than the normal size. At seventy years of age, my size will be increased by fifty percent of normal and at the age of eighty, I shall be bigger by eighty percent. My enlargement is both benign and malignant. Malignancy is not very common but God forbid, if I become cancerous, please cut me out of the body so that no other friend in my neighborhood becomes cancerous.

I am fifty years old now. During the last few years, my size and weight have increased and now the tissues surrounding me are also pressing me inwards. I cannot expand more due to lack of space and hence I have to press the urethra more. The wall of bladder, my friend, is getting thicker and irritable. Naturally, it is contracting even when it has very little quantity of urine. This makes me uncomfortable and my urine is frequent. I know I am causing scanty urination and I have to get up during the night and early morning to urinate. This is because my increased weight is pressing the urinary bladder. It is all right that you are tolerating this problem and trying to tone up the muscles of bladder and urethra through some 'Yoga' exercises. If my weight goes on increasing, you will have retention of urine, dribbling of urine, escape of semen after urination and you will feel as if some drops are left inside which you cannot vacate. At that time, it would be better if you get my photographs on ultrasound machine. Also get your blood urea, ESR and PSA examined.

At present I am having some problem with my health and I advice you to take me to a doctor. Thanks. Well, here comes the finger of the surgeon to feel me. The doctor has inserted his finger in your rectum to reach me. To him I felt hard but without any nodule. I am happy to hear that I am not to be disturbed and cut by a knife at present. But you should follow the directions of the doctor. Stop your tea, coffee, and intake of spicy and fried food. Over and above, do not have intercourse with your wife now onwards till the doctor tells you that I am in my normal condition. Another thing, please do not drink alcohol, which you used to consume every other day with your friends.

Here is a piece of advice. Whenever you feel that my passage has blocked and you are having difficulty in urinating, contact the doctor. He will pass a rubber tube through the urethra to the bladder. He can remove me if I am found too large. In other case, he will insert a small round instrument in the urethra and he can view the whole of inside. He can then cut the obstructing tissue through an electrically operated cutting loop. He may also freeze the blocking tissue with liquid nitrogen. I am just telling you all this so that you do not get afraid of some major surgery.

I shall advice you to start 'Yoga' and with it some homeopathic medicines to maintain my health and keep me in status quo. No medicine can shrink my size to normal. I am not going to bother you and shall be delivering you my efficient work without any hindrance from the pressed bladder.

I also request you to get my condition checked through rectal route twice every year from a doctor. If you find my condition deteriorated, be it benign or malignant, do not hesitate to get me expelled from your body. I do not mind if your body is saved and I am out of it. If you ever hesitate that upon my operation, you would go impotent, it is a wrong notion. Only one out of five patients undergoing surgery get impotent. There would not be any change in your sexual capacity.

Thank you for reading me.

Your most sincere gentle, genteel and genetic organ,

Prostate

DO YOU KNOW THE LOCATION OF YOUR PROSTATE GLAND?

- Have a look below the navel. There are pubic hair above the penis. Press here and you will feel an edge of bone beneath your pressing fingers of the right hand. This is the pubic bone.
- Now, move fingers of the left hand directly opposite to this pubic bone and press above the mid of two hips. You will feel presence of another bone. This is called the coccyx.
- Draw an imaginary straight line between the pubic bone and the coccyx. This line will cross and touch your prostate gland. At this very place, the urethra (excretory canal or tube of the bladder) is also located. The urine passes from the bladder through urethra.
- This urethra crosses the prostate gland. This means the prostate gland surrounds urethra in the same way as a ring surrounds and fits a finger.

ENLARGEMENT AND CANCER OF PROSTATE

- B.P.H. (Benign Prostatic Hypertrophy) or B.H.P. (Benign Hypertrophy of Prostate) or enlargement of prostate gland does not require any treatment until it produces symptoms.
- If you are 50 to 55 years of age, your urine frequency is more than usual during night and flow of urine falls vertically down without making an arc, it is time to get your prostate checked. (See page 43–self examination)
- *The symptoms of B.P.H. are:* frequent urination at night, weak flow of urine, discomfort during urination, incapability of holding back urine and great urge.
- Indian men have less frequency of prostatic enlargement in younger age group. In Negroes of Africa, prostatic enlargement is rare and in the Asiatic, it is exceptional.
- Postponement of urge for passing urine may lead to enlargement of prostate gland. (See page 26)
- B.H.P. takes many years to develop and it is wise to get a medical examination done as soon as the first symptoms appear.
- In the early stages of B.H.P., there is increased libido (desire to have sex), but in the later stages, impotence is the rule.

WHEN TO UNDERGO SURGERY FOR PROSTATE?

- Over four lakh men suffer from B.P.H. and over two lakh suffer from cancer of the prostate in U.S.A. It is the second most dangerous type of cancer in men that kills about forty thousand men each year in the U.S.
- Prostate gland is more susceptible to cancer than other organs of the human body.
- Indian males suffer from prostate cancer and still do not know it. Almost eighty percent of men aged more than sixty-five years have microscopic cancer of prostate. It takes decades to develop this cancer.
- B.P.H. can also convert to cancer of prostate if symptoms of cancer are neglected. (See page 32)

WHAT TO EAT AND WHAT NOT TO EAT FOR PROSTATE-CANCER PATIENTS? (SEE PAGE 105)

WHAT IS THE FIRST AID HOME TREATMENT FOR B.P.H. (SEE PAGE 67)

INFORMATION YOU WOULD LIKE TO KNOW ABOUT B.P.H. / B.H.P.

What is B.P.H. or B.H.P.?

B.P.H. is Benign Prostatic Hyperplasia or Hypertrophy as is known in USA. In India, some doctors name it B.H.P. or Benign Hypertrophy of Prostate. It is a condition wherein a man's prostate gland gets enlarged.

What are the symptoms of B.P.H.?

Some of the important symptoms that a man experiences due to BHP are:

- Frequent urination during night in particular.
- Difficulty in urinating.
- Painful or burning sensation during urination.
- Urine flow not easily stopped.

What are the causes of B.P.H.?

The main cause of B.P.H. is formation of dihydrotestosterone (DHT).

With the increasing age, say more than 45 or 50, the body converts more testosterone into DHT. (Testosterone is an androgen hormone and it stimulates bone and muscle growth and sexual development. It is produced in the testes).

What is the treatment available in India for B.P.H.?

The doctor tells the patient to keep a watch after he gives some primary medicines. If the patient feels that he is getting some relief in his symptoms, he should consult a doctor after 15 days.

Doctor may give some drugs to relax the muscles of the prostate and to block the hormones that enhances the prostatic growth or give medicines to relax the bladder to improve upon continence.

Surgery is the last resort. Depending on the condition, size and enlargement of the prostate and other related medical problems, the doctor decides which surgical procedure is best suited to the patient.

(See page 105 of this book for knowing how to care for your prostate gland.)

CONTENTS

SECTION - I

PROSTATE AND REPRODUCTIVE SYSTEM

In our ancient 'Vedas', 'Puranas' and religious books of Hindus, it is said that the body of human being comes after donning eighty four thousand creatures (Yoni). I am not aware whether this is true or not but one thing is sure that human body is an amazing creation of God that has everything including functioning, living, thinking and participating. It is like a society, a civilized society, in which every member participates, functions independently and yet collaboration is maintained so that the inside work and output are harmoniously done. There is a goal of living and welfare of each in society and it is true for the body organs. They function differently and yet contribute their achievements to achieve the goal. To do all this, there is a leader in the body as stands true in our society. It is the organizer or leader who guides and rules the body. The organizers and messengers in our body are *'hormones'* and the nervous system and the guidance is from the *brain.*

Hormones are chemical substances, which are the product of organs called endocrine glands. *'Endon'* means "within" and *'krinein'* means "to separate." The beauty is that the hormones pass directly into the blood stream without passing through a duct. There are some glands, which have a duct (salivary gland) and are called *exocrine glands.*

Hormones act in blood stream of the body but there are some hormones that have a limited action on one particular organ, called *target organ*. Endocrine glands like thyroid, parathyroid, adrenals, pancreas, gonads and pituitary are the better understood endocrine glands of the body. Prostate gland on the other hand is different in many ways. It comes under target organ category. We shall learn more about it later.

This small book is about the prostate gland but to know its location, purpose and functions, it is better if we start with other glands to understand what we ought to learn.

THE ENDOCRINE GLANDS

Endocrine is a Greek word that means *"internal secretion."* In our body, we have internal secretions and there is a complete endocrine system that works. The endocrine glands are ductless glands. They make a secretion but the secretion does not leave the glands by means of any duct. The secretion is passed into the blood, circulating through the substance of the gland. This vital principle of an internal secretion is called *hormone,* which means *'to excite'* (hormone is a Greek word). Some of our endocrine glands secrete single hormones whereas some others secrete two or more hormones. For example, Pituitary gland is secreting a number of hormones and it controls the activity of many other endocrine organs. On account of this activity of control, **Pituitary gland is called the 'master gland of the body'**.

Endocrine glands are made in a pattern following the glands of father and mother. In other words, it is the heredity that counts. The parents contribute to it at the time of conception. The formation of glands also depends upon the behavior and environmental changes in childhood. According to a view if the child is told too much of ghost stories or threatened time and again, his endocrine glands may get affected. Food and drinking water also affect the endocrine built and an example of this is the thyroid gland. In other cases occupation, pollution and lack of sunlight change the properties of secretions of glands. Infections also cause a tremendous changes in the glands.

Endocrine glands have a beautiful network and they control the body. Each of our glands is independent in its working, efficiency and output and still they depend upon each other for completion of an organ's work. This means they are interdependent too.

REPRODUCTIVE SYSTEM

Reproductive system is an apparatus working in all higher animals and human beings. In this system there is a genital, which is generally divided into the external and internal gentalia.

EXTERNAL GENTALIA

The topic of our book is prostate that belongs to males and hence we would talk about male's external genitalia only. In males, the genitals consist of the penis and the scrotum that is outside and a cutaneous sac is holding the testes and their epididymides. (Epididymis is a small body lying close to the posterior border of the seminal gland). The male genital system is designed to produce sperms and deposit them in the female. In action, the penis does this job.

Penis consists of a glans, a body and a root. The glans is the thickened distal end at the tip of which the urethra opens. Between the glans and the body is a narrow portion called the neck. The penis is covered with skin which forms folds called foreskin or prepuce on the glans. As the penis enlarges during erection, the foreskin peels back to leave the glans exposed to the stimulation, which leads to orgasm. The skin and the glans and the foreskin make a greasy substance called **smegma** that acts as a lubricant facilitating the movement of the foreskin over the glans. Young men in the family should be told to wash the glans regularly because in some men smegma tends to accumulate forming cheesy and smelly material that can cause soreness and inflammation of the foreskin. This condition called 'balanitis' might be a reason that people belonging to a particular sect carry out circumcision.

The root of penis is attached to the pubic bones. The penis has three so-called *corpora cavernosa* (cavernous bodies). Two of them are *corpora cavernosa* of the penis and one is the *corpus cavernosum* of the urethra because it transmits the urethra. The distal end of the corpus cavernosum urethrae is thickened and forms the glans penis. Each corpus cavernosum is covered with dense connective tissue coat and is of a spongy type structure. The numerous connective tissue septa form small cavities called caverns. The caverns fill with blood and the penis becomes turgid and erect during sexual excitement.

The male urethra therefore serves not only for voiding the urine from the bladder but also for ejaculating the seminal fluid. The urethra connects the bladder where urine is stored to a hole at the tip of penis (meatus). On the other hand, semen enters the urethra during intercourse through a pair of tubes called the seminal ducts or vas deferens which join it shortly after it leaves the bladder. A tight ring of muscles at the opening from the bladder into urethra keeps the passage closed so that urine only emerges when it is intended. The male urethra serves a double purpose of voiding the urine from the bladder and for ejaculating the seminal fluid. Urethra is about 16 to 18 cm in length and passes through the prostate, the urogenital diaphragm and the corpus cavernosum in the penis. We can say that it has three basic portions: prostatic, membranous and spongy portions. The **spongy or the penile portion** is the longest, say about 12 to 14 cm and it ends in the external orifice of the urethra in the glans penis. The posterior part of the spongy portion is dilated. This is called the bulbous part of the urethra. It is here that ducts of Cowper glands open. **Cowper gland** is one of the two glands located at the base of the prostate gland and on either side of the membranous urethra that produce a mucinous substance that lubricates the urethra and coats its surface. **The membranous portion** is the narrowest and shortest and measures about 1 cm and it is tightly fused with the urogenital diaphragm.

Out of these three portions, the **prostatic portion** is the widest. The length of it is about 3 cm. There is a swelling on its posterior wall called *seminal colliculus* (small mound). It is here where two ejaculatory ducts through which the seminal fluid is transmitted from the seminal glands and the ducts of the prostate gland meet. Secretions of prostate gland is a constituent of the seminal fluid. The distal part of the spongy portion lying exactly behind the external urethral orifice is also dilated. This is called the *navicular fossa*. (Fossa is a depression, mostly longitudinal). The mucous coat of the spongy portion has small depressions called lacunas.

We will now discuss about the **male urethra**. It has two sphincters, internal and external. (Sphincter is a muscular ring, which opens and closes the exit of a passage. Commonly known sphincters are pyloric sphincter and anal sphincter). Internal sphincter contracts involuntarily since it is composed of smooth muscle tissue and surrounds the urethra at the site where it leaves the bladder. The external sphincter is in the urogenital diaphragm around the membranous portion of the urethra. It contracts voluntarily since it is composed of striated muscle tissue. Male urethra has two curves called prepubic and subpubic. The prepubic curve is permanent whereas the subpubic curve straightens out upon the erection of the penis. When a catheter is introduced into the bladder, the structure and position of male urethra is always taken into account especially its constrictions, dilatations and curves.

INTERNAL MALE GENITALIA

The internal genitalia of man consists of two seminal glands (or two testes) and their appendages, the deferent and ejaculatory ducts, the seminal vesicles and the prostate and bulbo-urethal or Cowper's glands. Internal genitalia is abundantly supplied with nerves as is common with all internal organs. The internal genitalia of females consists of ovaries, uterus, uterine tubes and vagina. The complete system of testes in males and ovaries in females are also called 'gonads' although it is with the internal genitalia system. (Gonad means reproductive gland that produces sex hormones). During puberty, the gonads begin to grow and become active under the influence of the gonadotropic hormones that are the products of pituitary gland. These hormones stimulate the production of sex hormones, testosterones or androgens in males and estrogens and

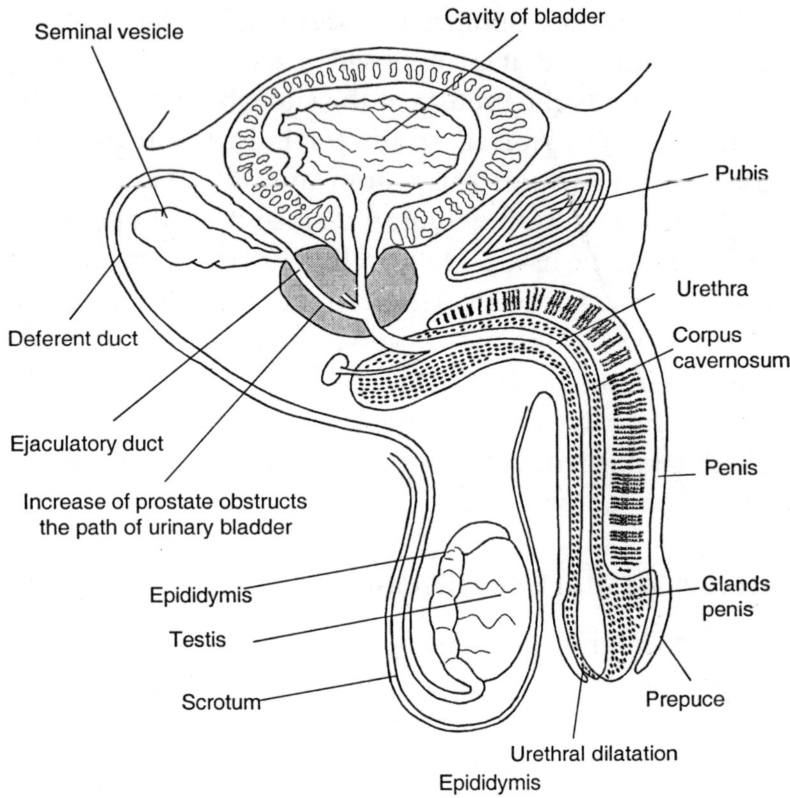

Fig. 1. Section of the Male Genitalia

progesterones in females. These sex hormones accelerate the growth of the genitalia as well as of secondary sexual characteristics like growth of larynx (change from mild childish voice to deep male voice) in the males and beginning of menstruation in females.

TESTES

The testis or orchis is one of the two male reproductive or seminal glands located in the scrotum. The function of testes is double. They provide the site where spermatozoa (male germ cells) multiply and male sex hormones 'testosterone' are manufactured. These two functions are carried out by separate sets of cells within each of the testis. Testis is an oval shaped body somewhat flattened at the sides. It has a covering of dense connective tissue membrane, which is called the tunica albuginea testis because of its color resemblance with cooked egg white. This connective tissue membrane forms a thickening at the posterior border of the testis and is called mediastinum testis. Connective tissue septa divides the testis into lobules. The lobules have thin tubes called convoluted tubules of the testis and its walls are made up of supporting and seminiferous cells. The seminiferous cells change by a series of complex transformations into spermatozoa. This process of transformation is called 'spermatogenesis'. Spermatozoa are found in fluid secretion and together they are the constituents of seminal fluid. The details of formation of seminal fluid are given because its discharge in sexual intercourse through the urethra includes the secretion of prostate and of the seminal vesicles. The sperm is delivered to the mediastinum testis from the seminiferous tubules. From here it travels to the duct of the epididymis.

The testis of the foetus is situated in the abdominal cavity and descends through the inguinal canal into the scrotum. By the time, the birth takes place both testes are usually in the scrotum. We have talked about epididymis above. Let us know about it.

Epididymis is a small body lying close to the posterior border of the seminal gland. It has a duct, which is continuous with the deferent duct.

The deferent duct is like a tube that is about 40-50 cm long and serves to transmit the seminal fluid. Its walls has three coats - mucous, muscular and connective tissue. The duct rises from the inferior end of the epididymis and enters the inguinal canal through its subcutaneous ring. In the inguinal canal, the deferent duct runs in the spermatic cord.

The spermatic cord has the thickness of the little finger and is composed of the different duct, nerves, blood and lymph vessels of the testis and of the epididymis. A common fascial membrane surrounds them. This means each testis is suspended in the scrotum by the spermatic cord. The deferent duct separates from the vessels and nerves at the deep ring of the inguinal canal. It descends into the cavity of the true pelvis and then to the fundus of the bladder. On the other hand, the blood and lymph vessels and nerves ascend towards the abdominal cavity. The deferent duct joins the excretory duct of the seminal vesicles near the prostate, thus forming the ejaculatory duct. The spermatic cord hence serves two purposes. It provides a blood supply to the testes and secondly, it conducts the newly formed sperm away from the testes.

The seminal vesicle is a paired organ of elongated form and is about 4 to 5 cm long. It is situated between the fundus of the bladder and the rectum. The seminal vesicles act as reservoirs for the seminal fluid. They also produce a secretion that is a constituent of this fluid.

Ejaculatory duct is formed above by junction of the deferent duct and the duct of the seminal vesicle. It passes through the substance of the prostate and opens into the prostatic part of the urethra. Ejaculatory duct discharges about 200 million sperms at each ejaculation.

Sperm

The male reproductive cell is called the sperm. It is made up of a number of chemicals and genetic material. The material is a chromosome, which carries the genetic blueprint of the father and this determines the paternally inherited characteristics of the child. The sperm also forwards the genetic message to determine the sex of the child.

Its only use is to achieve fertilization by union with the female cell, the ovum. Every sperm is about 0.008 mm in length and looks like a tadpole. It is the smallest of all human cells. It has three part's: a head, a mid section and a whip like tail about nine times as long. The front of the head contains special enzymes that can penetrate into the ovum for fertilization purpose.It appears to be charged with amazing store of energy that enables it to swim its way to the ovum. See the size of a sperm and its journey of about 12 cm up to the ovum. It is equal to a five mile upstream swim of a man. The mid section holds the vital source of energy required by the sperm on its journey to the ovum. The tail portion of the sperm is like a rocket. It propels the sperm to move like a whip with a speed of about 3mm per minute. The manufacture of sperm necessitates a temperature of about three degrees centigrade lower than the rest of the body. Hence, the manufacturing takes place within the scrotum. The surrounding tissue helps to regulate the temperature of the testicles inside the scrotum by pulling them upwards to the body in cold conditions and by a rich supply of blood vessels that dissipate the heat when the temperature gets too high. Sperm production is at the rate of ten to thirty billion a month. The beauty of the functioning of body is that in case of no ejaculation and no intercourse, the sperms disintegrate and are reabsorbed. When the sperms are ejaculated into the vagina of a woman, they move very fast so that they reach cervix and into the uterus speedily where they make their way into the fallopian tubes. It is here that fertilization may occur if an egg is present.

THE PROSTATE GLAND

We have read above that the Pituitary is the master gland of the body. In the same way, we can say that **prostate gland is the king gland**. It is only present in males, the kings and the females or the queens do not have it. Moreover, it has a definite role to create a race, the human race.

Prostate gland is a solid, English walnut-shaped organ that surrounds the first part of the urethra in the male. The prostate gland surrounds urethra in the same way as a ring surrounds a finger. Its location is under the bladder and in front of the rectum and it produces secretions that form part of seminal fluid during ejaculation. At the time of birth of male child, its weight is a few grams and its enlargement starts at the time of puberty. Near the age of twenty or so, its weight is 20 grams. A young man's

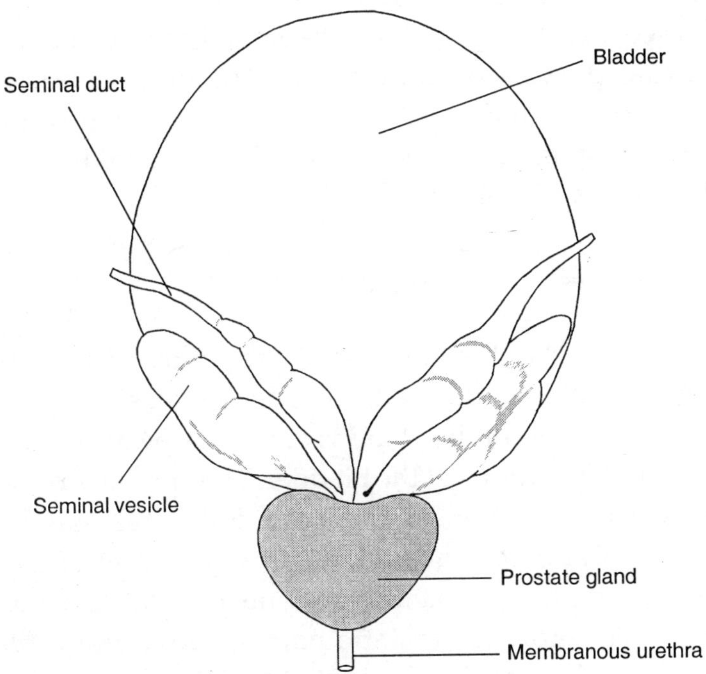

Fig. 2. Prostate Gland

prostate is of the size of a walnut, one and half inches in width, one inch in length and three fourth of an inch in thickness. In the later part of life, prostate gland is apt to increase in size and cause great difficulty in urinating. Sometimes, blood substitutes, precedes or follows urine, causing inflammation in whole of the bladder and sometimes it behaves like difficulties of climacteric as found in woman. Hypertrophy of prostate is compensatory to the warning of the function of testes. In India, according to some reports, 35% of men over sixty have an enlarged prostate. This enlargement means increased secretion, which has depraved action resulting in sexual perversion and mental disturbance. Since prostate comes under the reproductive system, it would be better if other related organs are also discussed here to make the anatomy clear.

ANATOMY

Prostate gland is situated in the cavity of the true pelvis under the fundus of the bladder and has a base and an apex. The base of the gland is directed upwards and is fused with the fundus of the bladder. The apex is directed downwards and adheres to the urogenital diaphragm. The prostate gland is made of muscular (smooth) and glandular tissue. The glandular tissue forms lobes whose ducts open into the prostatic part of the urethra. The secretion of the gland is a constituent of the seminal fluid as already said above. When the muscular tissue contracts, it helps the gland to empty the ducts and performs the function of urethral sphincter. It should be clear that the prostate gland gives passage to the urethra and the two ejaculatory ducts. In the old age, the gland gets enlarged due to increase in its connective tissue and it may interfere with the emptying of urinary bladder.

The prostate consists of glandular tissue embedded in a fibro-muscular stroma, surrounded by a fibrous capsule. It has the shape of the inverted triangle or is conical and presents for examination, a base and apex, a posterior, an anterior and two inferolateral surfaces. The base is directed upwards and is directly continuous with the neck of the urinary bladder. This is the reason it looks conical. The apex is directed downwards and is in contact with the superior fascia of the urogenital diaphragm. The posterior surface is separated from the rectum by fascia of Dennonvilliers (*rectovesicle septum*). These depressions serve to divide the posterior surface into lower larger and upper smaller portions. The upper smaller part is known as the *median lobe* whereas the lower larger portion is further divided by a shallow median groove, which separates this portion into right and left lateral lobes. These lobes are connected in front of urethra by a band, known as the *isthmus*, which is devoid of glandular substance. The anterior surface lies behind the symphysis pubis from which it is separated by prostatic plexus of veins and some loose fatty tissue. The inferolateral surfaces are related to the anterior parts of the levator ani muscle but are separated from this structure by a plexus of veins.

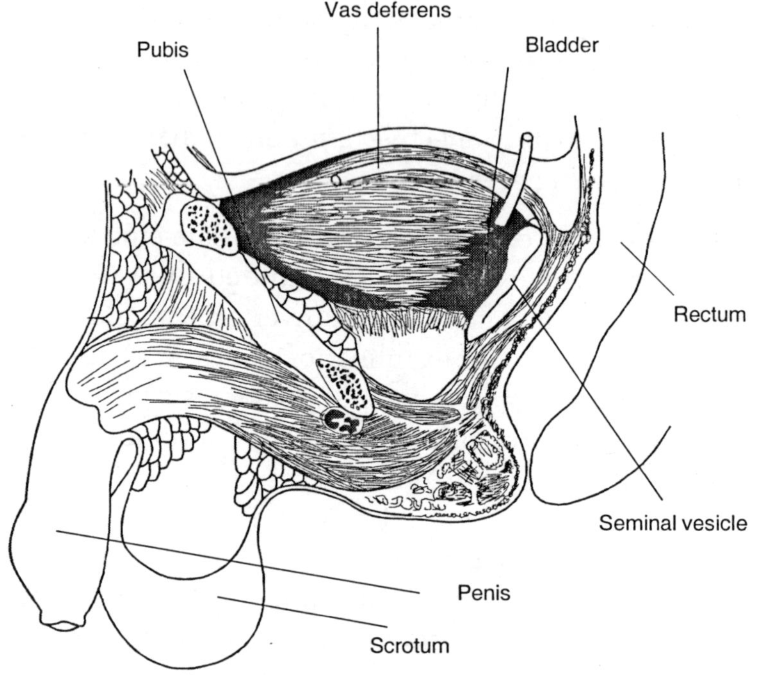

Fig. 3. Position of the Prostate

The prostate gland is divisible into five lobes. An anterior, middle and a posterior lobe and the two lateral lobes. The median lobe lies between the urethra in front and two common ejaculatory ducts behind. On either side of median lobe are the two lateral lobes, which extend backwards forming the posterior surface of the gland. These lobes are purely anatomical without any functional significance.

The posterior surface of the gland is directly related to the rectum and can be palpated during rectal examination.

GLANDS

There are three major types of glands in the prostate gland. These are: the **periurethral** glands, the **submucosal** glands and the **external** glands. Periurethral glands are the smallest and the other two form the largest portion of the prostate.

CELLS

There are two layers of cells: flat cuboidal (cells shaped resembling a cube) cells and tall columnar cells. Cuboidal cells are in the basal layer while tall columnar cells are faced towards the lumen of the gland. The glands are surrounded by an eosinophilic basement membrane.

EMBRYOLOGY

The prostate gland is made by evagination from the posterior urethra and hence can be called as belonging to endodermal origin. Endocrine stimulation causes normal development.

CONGENITAL ANOMALIES OF THE PROSTATE

Generally it is linked with malformations of the urogenital system. The prostate may, therefore, be **absent or smaller** than the usual size. In some cases, **abnormal growth** may develop in between the prostate and the ureter or urethra or both. In such an event, communications may form cavities termed as **diverticula** that resemble cysts in the prostate.

■

SECTION - II

CAUSATION-PATHOLOGY-EFFECTS-CLINICAL FEATURES & EXAMINATION OF PATIENT

BENIGN PROSTATE HYPERTROPHY (B.P.H.)

CAUSES

Prostatitis is the inflammation of prostate gland, caused mainly due to bacterial spread from urethra. Presence of urinary catheterization may also be one of the reason for prostatitis. Here are the opinions of different schools.

RIGIDITY AND OLD AGE

Many doctors believe that prostatitis or enlargement of prostate is not an affliction of a particular organ or a local illness. It is due to rigidity that starts to reveal its sphere in different parts of the body in old age. This rigidity means arteriosclerosis. The bladder and prostate gland also become rigid and hard. On the other hand, there is a different view by some doctors. They say that prostate gland enlargement has been noticed in those old men who have no signs of arteriosclerosis. This makes the earlier statement controversial.

Old age has two distinct problems: *rigidity of joints* and *cataract in the eyes.* The third problem, unknown to most of the people in their old age, is the complaint of urine that manifests itself in many ways. Sometimes it passes with interruption and by drops and the man has to wait for a longer time to finish the act of urination and at times it is accompanied by a burning sensation. It is very troublesome, inconvenient and uncomfortable for an old man to get up during night and early morning to urinate six or seven times. This happens when there is disease of prostate.

EXCESSIVE SEXUAL INDULGENCE

A school of opinion thinks that enlargement of prostate gland is due to excessive sexual indulgence. Men who are always thinking about sex/dwell upon sex, men who make various fantasies of sexual intercourse or men who see a woman on the road or in a picture and make love in imagination, are prone to this disease in their old age.

GONORRHEA

Gonorrhea is a gonococcal infection arising from impure sexual intercourse. In Hindi, it is called 'Parmeh' or 'sujak'. Those men who visit prostitutes frequently are prone to get this infection. According to a view, gonorrheal infection attacks the urinary tract and spreads to urethra and then to prostate. Prostate is inflamed and enlarged due to this.

MASTURBATION

Masturbation is also supposed to lead to prostatitis and enlargement of prostate. The reason attributed by some doctors for this act of masturbation is that the prostate has to force frequent fluid although there are no exact accessories like natural stimulation and release of natural sex hormones.

PROSTATE AND UTERUS

According to another view of some doctors, there is a resemblance between uterus and prostate. There is tumor formation in the uterus in middle or old age in women and it is natural. Similar is the case with enlargement of prostate. Tumor in the uterus grows when a woman is not much indulging in sexual activities. Enlargement of prostate also starts when the sexual activities of men are on the decline. This means that both the complaints start in men and women when their sexual power is on the decline. It does not start when the sexual power of both men and women is completely gone. This means that there is some relation between enlargement of the prostate and the sexual power of man.

POSTPONEMENT OF URINE

I have seen people in the office or in the market or travelling in the bus who postpone the urge to urinate due to no toilet available or are hesitant to urinate in the open. Similarly there are people who are lazy and hesitate to go for urination although there is an urge for it. This may lead to prostatic troubles irrespective of the age of the person. Postponing the urge to pass urine exerts pressure on the bladder. The bladder has a limited space to expand, beyond which it cannot inflate. The result is that the pressure of urine and its retention in the bladder makes the walls of bladder thick, especially at the neck. This pressure is transmitted to the prostate gland through urethra and compresses the gland. Compression means widening of the area. After all, the prostate gland is like a ring around the urethra. This ring expands due to compression. Expansion means enlargement. If the urge for urination is suppressed time and again, the prostate gland goes on expanding by and by.

CONCLUSION ON THE ABOVE VIEWS

The above explained reasons are only views and they do not appear to be justified except the reason of old age. One can object to them and raise the following questions:

- Why people do not have enlargement of the prostate gland when they are actually engaged in masturbation, sexual acts and excesses and sighting or fantasizing about sex during the youth?
- Why young persons suffering from gonorrhea are not found with enlarged prostate?
- If the reasoning as above is correct, the increase of prostate should occur when these activities are being indulged in.
- How is it that this problem comes up in old age when the men have left all those activities undertaken in young age.

A reason in support of this contention is that the urine does not pass easily soon after the coition. It shows that prostate gland gets enlarged temporarily after the sexual act. Excessive repeated sexual acts, therefore, could be a reason for enlargement of prostate.

In fact, the body in young age is flexible and it is the rigidity of the body that can be one reason for enlargement of prostate. The reason of rigidity of body in old age was the conclusion of French doctors and it appears to be rational. One notices the rigidity in all parts of the body in old age and prostate is also a part of body and hence liable to become rigid. Rigidity means non-elasticity, which means increase of weight. This is what happens to prostate. It is rigidity that brings cataract, arthritis, and rheumatism, freezing of body parts and backache.

Benign enlargement of the prostate normally occurs after the age of fifty years by Indian standards. It is most often between sixty and seventy years of age. According to 'The short book of surgery' by Bailey and Love, Indian men have less frequency of prostatic enlargement and it occurs more often in a younger age group. In Negroes of Africa, prostatic enlargement is rare and in Asiatic, it is exceptional. I am not sure about Negroes and Asiatic but the picture has really changed so far as India is concerned.

I have personally viewed many cases of prostate enlargement during my thirty-five years of practice and made adequate number of enquiries from my doctor friends both from homeopathy and allopathy. I have not found cases of young men suffering from this disease although the medical literature in western countries record that BHP is more found in younger age in India.

Regarding postponement of urine at the time of urge, the theory appears rational. No one can deny this theory. A pressure on the bladder due to voluntary retention exerts pressure on urethra, which in turn expands the surrounding prostate gland. It is also the postponement of urine urge that leads to retention of urine, total obstruction in the passing of urine or its passing with interruption, sometimes drop by drop and with burning sensation or pain. We have experienced such cases. No impulses of the body are to be obstructed. Retention of passing of urine when there is an urge may lead to enlargement of prostate especially in old men. (Please see 'do not stop these urges' on page 56)

ESTABLISHED THEORIES OF CAUSATION

Now we come to established theories of benign enlargement of prostate. There are two established theories of causation of benign enlargement of the prostate.

THE HORMONIC THEORY

One has to consider that hormonal influence has a definite role. Two testicular hormones govern the prostate; one is male (androgenic) and the other is female (estrogen). Normally the preponderant testicular hormone is the androgen that is supplemented by androgens secreted by the adrenal gland. Estrogen causes retrogressive changes in the testes and prostate gland.

It is a natural tendency that male hormones diminish with the advance of age while the quantity of the estrogenic hormone is not decreased equally or proportionately. This means that prostate enlarges due to predominance of the estrogenic hormone. Enlargement of prostate can be taken as involutionary hyperplasia akin to fibro-adenosis of the breast in women because of disturbance of the ratio and quantity of the circulating androgens and estrogens.

THE NEOPLASTIC THEORY

According to this theory, the enlargement of prostate is a benign neoplasm. [Neoplastic is relating to neoplasm. Neoplasm is a new growth comprised of an abnormal collection of cells, the growth of which exceeds and is uncoordinated with that of the normal tissues.

Neoplastic theory is about enlargement of glands of benign category that is for longer duration.] As the prostate is composed essentially of fibrous tissue, muscle tissue and glandular tissue, the neoplasm is a fibromyoadenoma. [Fibro is pertaining to fibre, myo is a prefix indicating muscle and fibromyoadenoma is muscular benign growth. Fibroadenoma is a benign tumor commonly found in breasts of young girls.]

Important note

The actual cause of BPH is not known so far and the above description is of possible causes only. The hormone theory is believed to be the one that is nearest to the causation.

PATHOLOGY

APPEARANCE

The enlarged prostate gland is rubber like and firm in consistency. Enlarged prostate weighs more than 50 gm whereas its normal weight is between 20 to 30 gm. There will be enlargement of middle lobe. If the posterior lobe is affected, it may be a case of prostate cancer. On cut section, the prostate may reveal numerous closely packed nodules exuding small amounts of milky fluid. Cystic changes may be present. The nodules are mostly granular while tissue is yellowish pink. It is demarcated and soft. The nodules are primarily fibromuscular and the tissue is yellowish gray. It is not soft but tough and less demarcated.

Histologic appearance (Histology is microscopic study of the structure and functions of tissue. Histological appearance of the nodules vary and depends upon whether the nodules consists of only glandular structure or, equal amounts of glandular and stromal elements. It also depends upon whether nodules are predominantly smooth muscles and connective tissue.

Hyperplasia (increase in the number of cells in an organ). It is usually accompanied by hypertrophy or enlargement of the organ. Hyperplasia affects the glandular elements and connective tissue but in variable degree. Benign adenomatous hyperplasia also affects the submucous group of glands resulting in or forming a nodular enlargement. This enlargement is mostly of lateral lobes that compresses the external group of glands into a false capsule. With the enlargement of prostate, there is a tendency to displace seminal vesicles. The result is that instead of lying on the base of the bladder, these structures become a direct posterior relation of the upper limit of the prostate. When the hyperplasia affects the subcervical glands, there is development of a middle lobe. This lobe projects up into the bladder with the internal sphincter. Many a times, both the lateral lobes get projected into the bladder. In such a case, the sides and back of the internal urinary meatus look surrounded by an intravesicle prostatic collar. One can compare BPH as approaching of menopause for males as are the complications in the menopause of females. We have already stated while studying hormonic theory that in males, the ratio of testosterone to estrogen is active while in females this ratio is increased. The male hormone testosterone is at the high when the male is in his adolescence. It goes on decreasing with increase of age and at the age of about fifty years, it is quite low. To compensate this low level of testosterone, the body releases some other stimulating hormones. Such an act does not fulfill the demand of testosterone but it is now transformed into DHT (5-alpha-dehydro-testosterone). This DHT is the actual culprit that enlarges the size of prostate. Some research scholars do not agree with this theory.

EFFECTS OF PROSTATIC ENLARGEMENT

There are naturally some effects of benign prostate hypertrophy or enlargement of prostate in the body when the disease is ignored. Here are some of them:

1. ON BLADDER

Within the bladder, bands of muscle fibers can be seen. This is known as trabeculation of the bladder due to prostatic obstruction. (Trabicula is a bundle of connective tissue that subdivides an organ). Between the hypertrophied bundles, there are shallow depressions called sacculations. Sometimes, one of the saccules continues to enlarge and forms a diverticulum. The problem comes when the middle lobe swells upwards into the bladder, it acts as a storing tank for the last ounce or more of urine that remains in the post-prostatic pouch. When this standing urine becomes stagnant, there is a possibility to form calculi. It is natural that the residues of urine settle down and form a thick layer ultimately turning into stones.

Enlarged prostate may compress or push the prostatic venous plexus and the veins at the base of the bladder get congested and are likely to cause hematuria.

2. ON URETHRA

The part of the urethra that lies lying above the verumontanum (Colliculus seminalis) gets elongated and this elongation becomes double the original size sometimes. This results in compression of canal laterally so that it tends to become an antero-posterior slit. The normal posterior curve may be so aggravated that it needs a fully curved metal catheter to negotiate it. Lateral distortion of the prostatic urethra is bound to be there when one lateral lobe is enlarged.

3. ON URETERS AND KIDNEYS

Direct or indirect pressure of intravesicle portion of the prostate on the ureteric orifices mostly cause dilatation of the ureters. This is a gradual process but results in some degree of bilateral hydronephrosis. When bladder hypertrophy decreases, the sphincter mechanism around the ureteric orifices stop to function. The result is that there is reflux of urine from the bladder into the dilated ureters and this means increased damage to the renal parenchyma. This type of ascending infection gives rise to pyelonephrosis.

4. ON SEXUAL ORGANS

In early stages of prostate enlargement, there is increased libido. In later stages, impotance is the rule.

SYMPTOMS OF B.H.P. (ENLARGED PROSTATE)

BPH produces symptoms only in a small percentage of affected persons. This is the major reason why people come at a stage when acuteness of the disease calls for immediate action. When symptoms occur, they are the **secondary effects related to compression of the urethra** with the result that urine flow from the bladder is stopped. These two problems further deteriorate the condition of patient when he complaints of distension and hypertrophy of the bladder. Prostatitis, hydronephrosis, hydroureter, cystitis, renal infections, calculi and tuberculosis are identified in the later stage or already exist. In the views of most of the doctors, hypertrophy does not predispose to prostatic cancer.

There is a variation in the presentation of clinical features that depends upon the lobes affected. However, some important symptoms of the disease are listed below:

FREQUENCY OF URINE

One of the earliest symptoms of enlargement of prostate is frequency of urination. *In the start,* it is nocturnal and the patient is obliged to get up to micturate during the second part of sleep, i.e. after midnight, say by 2AM to 3AM. This frequent urination is on account of vesicle introversion of the sensitive prostatic mucous membrane. This happens due to intravesicle enlargement of prostate. The frequency of urination gradually increased becomes even during daytime. Due to enlargement of the prostate, there is stress on the vesicle sphincter and a little quantity of urine escapes into the normally empty prostatic urethra. This brings a sort of emergency, a reflex action, to empty the bladder. Mind it, this is in addition to the frequent voiding of urine. *In the later stage,* when the residual urine increases, frequency becomes more and more. This is the main reason why the urine dribbles. Further, in the event of neglect, when no treatment is taken, frequency is encouraged by cystitis (lower urinary tract infection-descending infection from kidney to adjacent structures) and polyurea (excessive urine frequency) due to renal insufficiency.

URINE STREAM

The stream of urine becomes variable. It is often weak and tends to stop and start and dribble towards the end of micturition.

In many cases, the urine falls vertically without any force. Normally, the flow of urine should appear like an arc and not vertical.

DIFFICULT MICTURITION

There is a 'wait' for the patient to start urination and it requires some time. Even straining for urine does not bring about the urine and the patient has to wait.

PAIN DURING OR AFTER URINATION

There is pain due to cystitis or acute retention of urine. When hydronephrosis commences, there may be dull pain in the loins. One feels a weight in the perineum (the floor of pelvis or space between the anus and scrotum or urethral opening) or fullness in the rectum.

ACUTE RETENTION OF URINE

Acute retention of urine is the most important symptom. The patient is so afraid that he immediately contacts the doctor to obtain relief from the pain that accompanies the retention of urine. The main causes of retention of urine are postponement of micturition at the time of urge and indulgence in alcoholic liquors due to which congestion of internal organs occur. If the patient is suffering from some illness and is on the bed, then also retention of urine may occur. Similarly after some surgical operation and confinement, urine retention is a possibility.

RETENTION OF URINE WITH OVERFLOW

In this condition, there is swelling due to distended bladder and no pain but urine constantly dribbles.

HAEMATURIA

Haematuria is a condition where the patient finds a drop of blood at the beginning or end of urination. If there is a ruptured prostatic vein or there is erosion of the enlarged prostate, bleeding to an alarming extent may occur. Such a condition when the bleeding is due to rupture of an enlarged prostate should be treated at the earliest. This condition of the prostate has been termed as 'decoy' prostate by some doctors.

RENAL INSUFFICIENCY

With enlarged prostate, when there is suppression of urine and the excretion is less than 300 ml of urine in twenty four hours (a condition called anuria) and hematuria is also reported, the case has to be dealt with separately for treatment of anuria. Renal insufficiency, in most of the cases, is not considered as the outcome of prostate enlargement.

SYMPTOMATIC CHARACTERISTICS OF B.H.P.

The enlargement of prostate (Benign Hypertrophy of Prostate or BHP) does not occur overnight and it takes years. It comes up gradually and has certain phases.

FIRST PHASE

There is a peaceful progression of the enlargement of prostate by the age of fifty or so and the patient does not know when it started enlarging, because there are not much symptoms. At times, patient has more frequency of urine and he does not care about it. He thinks this may be due to excessive intake of water on that day. In winters, he thinks that the water taken has no outlet like sweating and hence urine frequency is increased. In summers, if the urine dribbles or it is of less quantity with less frequency, he attributes it to summer and excessive sweating. He tries domestic medicines like 'saunf' or 'jeera' or some digestive tablets and feels comfortable. After a day or two, the problems of urine are over. If there is burning during urination, he consults a doctor and takes some medicines which provides symptomatic relief. No one thinks that he is nearing or above fifty years of age and that he should get his prostate checked. Such awareness is not there in Indian males. In U.S.A, this awareness is very much existent and even some prostate institutes are made where periodical checks can be undertaken.

So, in the very first stage, the problems are as above and are almost negligible. The patient gets more of urge for urination and his frequency of urination increases by two to three times more than his earlier habit or usual habit. As stated in above paragraph, the patient gets burning in urine and sometimes he has to wait for urine to start. He feels that the flow of urine from the penis is not having the pressure that he used to have earlier. But all these symptoms are temporary and do not persist for long. When the patient starts walking and moving, the urine passes without delay. If he continues to lie on the bed for long or sits watching TV or reads a book while lying down, he feels delay in urination but movement for sometime clears the urination. His urge for urination during the night is more but he does not bother. **The wonderful thing about this first state of prostate**

enlargement is that there is no big quantity of residual urine and the patient is still able to empty his bladder clearly. These symptoms come and go but the patient feels no need to consult a doctor. It is natural. Some times, we have constipation or diarrhea and home remedies or diet clears them and by the time one thinks of consulting a doctor, the disorder is gone. Such symptoms are, therefore, dealt with as disorders and not disease. Here lies the **first carelessness** on the part of patient in dealing with BHP. The first stage of BHP thus continues for several years.

SECOND PHASE

After suffering for years, the symptoms start appearing to show that enlargement of prostate has actually occurred. The new symptom is that the patient has to rise to urinate in the early morning say 4 to 5 A.M. while his usual time of getting up was 6 to 7 A.M. The pressure compels him to get up from bed but when he goes to the toilet, he finds the flow to be slow and the stream less forcible. One thing is to be made clear here. There are persons who take a glass of milk or take a glass or two of water before going to bed. They also get this habit of urinating in the early morning. The difference between the BHP and normal urination is that person with normal flow of urine will have the urge and when he goes to toilet, the urine is flushed out immediately. In the case of persons having BHP, the person goes to the toilet but finds the stream of urine slow and less forcible although his bladder is distended. He is inclined to strain but without success. (It may be noted that straining sometimes result in prolapse of rectum or may induce piles.)

And the strange point is that the urine escapes involuntarily when he thinks that he has completed the urination act. He waits for the urine to start but without any success. This is the **second phase.** (Read how to tone bladder muscles at this stage on page 67- first aid treatment)

THIRD PHASE

There is a universal notion and understanding about diseases. And this understanding is that there is no need to consult a doctor if there are no symptoms. If everything is going fine according to one's routine work and output, why to consult a doctor? The same stands good for BHP. There is no treatment needed unless it produces symptoms. It has been noticed that old and retired persons prone to enlargement of prostate gland do not get much of symptoms or do not bother about irregular and disordered urination until they find some compelling symptoms for consulting the doctor. This happens with those persons who have busy schedule of social or domestic work even after retirement. They are so busy that such disorders do not bother them and even if they are bothered, they resort to domestic herbs or 'yoga' by which they get slight relief. Slight relief does not mean that the prostate has not enlarged. It has enlarged but the attitude of the patient towards his body is so casual that he does not care much. I salute to such persons who do not care much about slight problems of the body. Most of the persons in old age make a hue and cry when they do not get their stools or are slightly disposed.

Let us come back to the third stage of enlargement of prostate. When the prostate swells enough to compress the urethra, which passes through it, it will obstruct the urine flow. This can lead to a desire to urinate day and night and on the other hand, the flow of urine becomes increasingly slow and hesitant. The patient is unable to pass urine except in small amount yet he suffers from incontinence.

As a result of the enlargement of prostate, the residual urine begins to collect in the bladder. This is **third phase of the disease**. The symptoms of the disease remain the same as faced in the first phase but they aggravate and start troubling the patient. Instead of going to toilet two times at night, now he goes to bathroom six to seven times in all during whole of night. On the other hand, the pain also starts in the lower abdomen i.e. bladder area due to swelling. The urge to urinate increases. While the pain in the first stage is occasional, in the second stage, it is frequent. Sometimes, the patient does not want to leave the bathroom thinking that some urine is still to come.

FOURTH PHASE

Third phase means increased frequency of urination. Now the family members of the patient also observe that the patient is not leaving the toilet spare for them to use. This frequent urination is due to vesicle introversion of the sensitive prostatic mucous membrane. This happens due to intravesicle enlargement of prostate. The frequency of urination is increase even during the daytime. Due to enlargement of the prostate, there is stress on the vesicle sphincter and a little quantity of urine escapes into the normally empty prostatic urethra. This brings a sort of emergency, a reflex action, to empty the bladder. Mind it, this is in addition to frequent voiding of urine. As a matter of fact, the enlargement of prostate gland takes place from all sides including bladder side in the back, urethral side in the front and from above to below because the urethra is completely covered all around by prostate gland. When this enlargement is all around, **it is the fourth phase** of disease and one has to urinate every hour or half an hour. In this stage, there may be either swelling at the opening of the bladder or obstruction of urine due to enlargement of bladder.

On increased frequency of urine, Dr. Satyavrata Siddhantalankar has cited a wonderful explanation. 'Suppose there is no enlargement of prostate and bladder collects 50 ounce of urine in 24 hours and further suppose there is a scope of passing only 10 ounces of urine at a time. This means that one expels urine five times in 24 hours. Now suppose the enlargement of prostate has occurred with the same person and 50 ounce of urine is collected in the bladder. Now there is obstruction at urethra and it allows only 6 to 8 ounces of urine to pass instead of 10 ounces. It means the same person has to urinate seven to eight times during the period. There will be some residual urine left in the bladder that can damage the bladder in the long run' (Courtesy book: From old age to youth through yoga).

When the residual urine increases, frequency becomes more and more. This is the main reason why the urine dribbles. Further, in the event of neglect when no treatment is taken, frequency is encouraged by cystitis (lower urinary tract infection-descending infection from kidney to adjacent structures) and polyurea (excessive urine frequency) due to renal insufficiency.

Now is the time to think about surgical operation of prostate.

EXAMINATION OF PATIENT

(A) SELF EXAMINATION

There are many complaints of prostate and all cannot be detected or examined by the patient himself. This book is to help those patients who are aware of the disease, have read somewhere about it or have been to doctor who told them the possibility of enlargement of prostate but has not checked the rectum. Besides the enlargement, the prostate gland can have cancer, which can be detected by a specialist. Here is a preliminary self-examination of prostate for the patient to observe or conduct.

Check urine flow: Hold the penis; draw the foreskin upwards so that the glans (distal end of the shaft of penis) is free to urinate. Now observe the flow of urine. It should be with force and fall on the ground in an arc. If it falls vertically without force on the ground, suspect prostatic trouble.

Note the frequency of urine: There is a link between the frequency of urine, intake of water, the amount of sweating, exertion by the body and nature of work of a person. A normal person of 50 to 55 years of age has the urge to go for urination three to five times in a day and probably no urination during night after sleep. Prostatic trouble can be suspected if the person starts getting up during night for urination once or twice and the day urine frequency also increases and goes up to six or seven times. **In fact a change in frequency and quantity of urine flow more or less than normal indicates prostate problem.** Normal has different meaning for each individual. A man drinking 10 glasses of water and a man drinking five glasses of water will have different norms for urination. Any change in the urination timing, speed and quantity is abnormal if the change is noted after the age of about 50 to 55 years. One should consult the doctor at the earliest..

Check these Symptoms

In a nut shell, the symptoms of B.P.H are *frequent urination, urination at night and early morning, weak stream of urine, uncomfortable urination, incapability of holding back urine and great urge,* decreased libido and sexual performance. Now this is the time that a consultation with doctor is due.

(B) EXAMINATION BY DOCTOR

The prime method of examining the enlargement of prostate is rectal examination.

1. **Rectal examination** is generally done to locate any growth. Anal canal is approximately 2.5 cm long and is bordered by external and internal sphincters which are normally firm and smooth. Rectal examination is done to know the anatomical situation of internal piles and prostate. In the case of prostate, it is done bimanually (using both the hands) one hand on the hips and the other in the rectum. In benign enlargement of the lateral lobes, increase in their size is felt. The lobes appear smooth, convex and typically

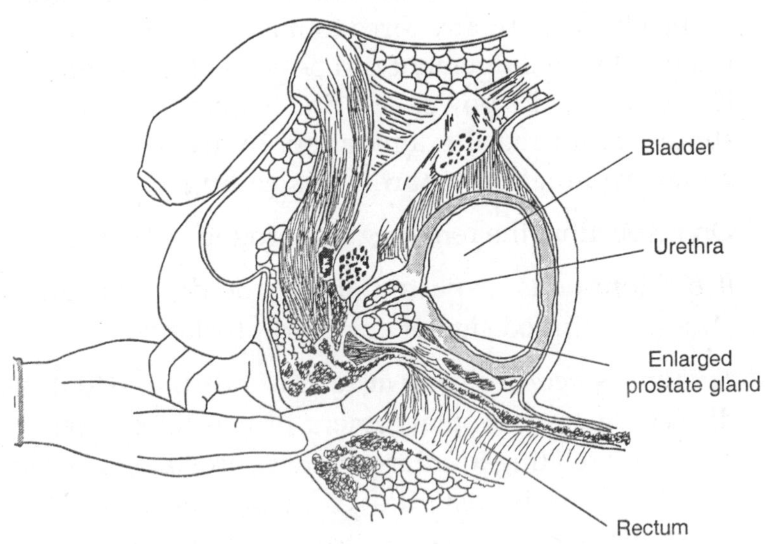

Fig. 4. Rectal Examination

elastic but the fibrous element may give the prostate a firm consistency. The rectal mucosa can be made to move over the prostate. On bimanual palpation, an intravesicle lobe can be felt. A pressure should be exerted on the apex of the prostate by inserting a finger in the rectum. One can find that the enlarged gland has a definite degree of mobility. Residual urine may be felt a fluctuating swelling above the prostate. There is enough amount of residual urine present and it pushes the prostate downwards, which is felt at larger than it is. This slight enlargement has to be kept in consideration. An expert surgeon or doctor having experience of rectal examination knows this fact. The bladder is not felt full.

The patient can be asked to tell about the projected flow of urine during urination. If the urine falls vertically without any force to make the flow an arc, the prostate enlargement can be predicted. After this loss of projectile power of urine is noted, the doctor should go for rectal examination. **In many cases, the rectal examination report is misleading.**

2. On inspection, the renal region is found to be **tender.**
3. If the **tongue** is inspected, it may be dry or brown. (Not a confirmed sign of enlarged prostate)
4. There is a **scoring system** to find out the extent of disease in case of enlargement of prostate. A set of questions relating to enlargement of prostate has been framed. This is just like you read self-assessing questionnaires in magazines to check your intelligence, obesity, digestion, condition of eyes etc.

In the case of prostate, you are asked to tell about your experience *in the past one month* about:

a. Frequency of urine.

b. Incomplete emptying of bladder.

c. Dribbling (intermittent).

d. Urge or urgency.

e. Forceless stream of urine.

f. Straining for urine.

g. Urine frequency during night (nocturnal).

All these points are given marks, say, if it is 'no', less than five times in the past one month, the mark is 1 and so on for each of the topic under 'a' to 'g'. All these marks from a to g are added and more the marks more the enlargement. This method is quite vague because the Indian man has a tendency to show that he is healthy even in old age and he does note prefer to undergo any treatment or operation. So, he might answer incorrectly, either deliberately or he may be genuinely not sure how to answer properly.

PATHOLOGICAL TESTS

- 'Ultrasound' is the first preference of all the doctors in small or big cities.
- The examination of rectum is also done by **Cystoscopy.** For this, an instrument called the 'cystroscope' is used. This gives a reliable information of the disease.

- When operation of prostate is imminent, doctors resort to **cysto-urethroscopy.** It is an essential preliminary to prostatectomy when the operation is not transvesical. This test reveals the presence of any growth, diverticulum or non-opaque stones. It would also ascertain whether there is urethral stricture or bladder neck obstruction. This examination is also essential if there is history of hematuria.
- Examination of blood for **blood urea** estimation, a **blood count** (WBC 5000-10,000/cu mm is normal) and Wassermann reaction are all-important. **Blood urea** (normal is 25-40 mg per cent) and **ESR** (0-15 mm per hour is normal) will be increased.
- Excretory **pyelography** is conducted to estimte find out renal function. It is omitted only if the patient shows clinical signs of renal failure or if the blood urea is high.
- **Prostate Specific Antigen (PSA)** test: It isa protein developed by the cells of the prostate gland. This test finds out the level of PSA in blood. Generally PSA level is low in men but in the case of benign or cancerous condition of prostate, PSA level is found to be increased. PSA level alone does not give sufficient information to confirm benign or cancerous prostate. (PSA level below 4 mg/ml is normal.)
- **IVU** is undertaken to ascertain the shape and position of urethra.
- **Urine flow test**: There is a special type of instrument and the patient is told to urinate. It will measure how

slow or quick is the urine- flow. A reduced urine flow is an indicator of BPH.

- **Pyelogram** will confirm or exclude the presence of hydroureters and hydronephroses. It can also be used to know vesicle diverticulums. If the film is taken after micturation, one can know the amount of residual urine.
- **Radiological evidence** (X-ray) is one of the best methods to ascertain the complete picture of residual urine.
- **Color Doppler and tissue hormonic ultrasound** is useful for fluid filled organs.
- **Endorectal MRI** is also undertaken in many cases.

Some times **bone scan** is essential along with update on prostate CT and MRI fusion.

METHODS OF TREATMENT OF B.H.P. WITH OR WITHOUT SURGERY

In case of retention of urine, your doctor in the neighborhood would immediately put you to **catheterization**. This is the first step treatment. (Read more about it step wise in the heading 'prostatectomy').

TUMT AND TUNA

When catheterization is not very effective, TUMT, is undertaken, TUMT is *Transurethral Microwave*

Thermotherapy. There is a device called Prostratron that destroys the excessive prostate tissues. It is a complicated procedure. While the computer regulated microwave sends heat signals, the other part of the machine cools the urethra so that there is no damage done. This test is available in big hospitals. TUMT does not help reduce the hypertrophy although it may reduce urinary urgency, frequency, retention, straining etc. to some extent. TUNA is *Transurethral Needle Ablation*. TUNE works on the same principle of burning a well defined aea of prostate. The heat is generated through low level radio frequency energy. It has the same limitations as that of TUMT and prostate enlargement is not corrected. TUNA is *Transurethral Needle Ablation.*

TRANSURETHRAL SURGERY (TURP)

Who is the patient preferring to get cured for retention of urine or other connected problems and undergo TUMT or TUNA? Even doctors would not advice the said costly methods which do not serve the purpose permanently i.e. enlargement of prostate. If the enlargement is not very great, Transurethral surgery is preferred by doctors and patients alike in almost 90 percent of the cases. The reason is that Prostate has been considered a gland concerning the sexual capability (?) wrongly or rightly by men and no man will desire to get the prostate removed totally. I am not talking of USA and other developed countries where people have the means to go in for experiments and wait for results. The word TURP is *Transurethral Resection of Prostate.* An instrument called 'resectoscope' is inserted in the hole of penis. Through this instrument the tissues are act with the help of electrical loop and the blood vessels are sealed. The wire-loop attached to the instrument removes the tissue ends one at a time. The cut pieces are carried to the bladder via fluid and at the end of operation, they are flushed out.

LASER SURGERY

It is a surgical procedure that makes the use of laser fiber to vaporize the obstructing tissue. Laser fiber is inserted into the urethra with the help of a cystoscope and laser energy beams are then passed for a few seconds. The laser beams destroy the enlarged prostate tissue and shrinks it. This type of laser exposure is not very common and its side effects are not known so far. It is not an open surgery but the patient is anesthetized.

PROSTATECTOMY (SURGICAL OPERATION OF PROSTATE)

It is an open surgery where an external incision is given. When the gland is greatly enlarged and there are associated urinary complications due to this enlargement, then this procedure is undertaken.

About thirty to forty percent of the patients who come for prostatectomy are compelled to go in for this operation because of acute or chronic retention of urine. The treatment for such cases is that patients with good general health, having no clinical signs of infection or renal insufficiency should undergo immediate one stage

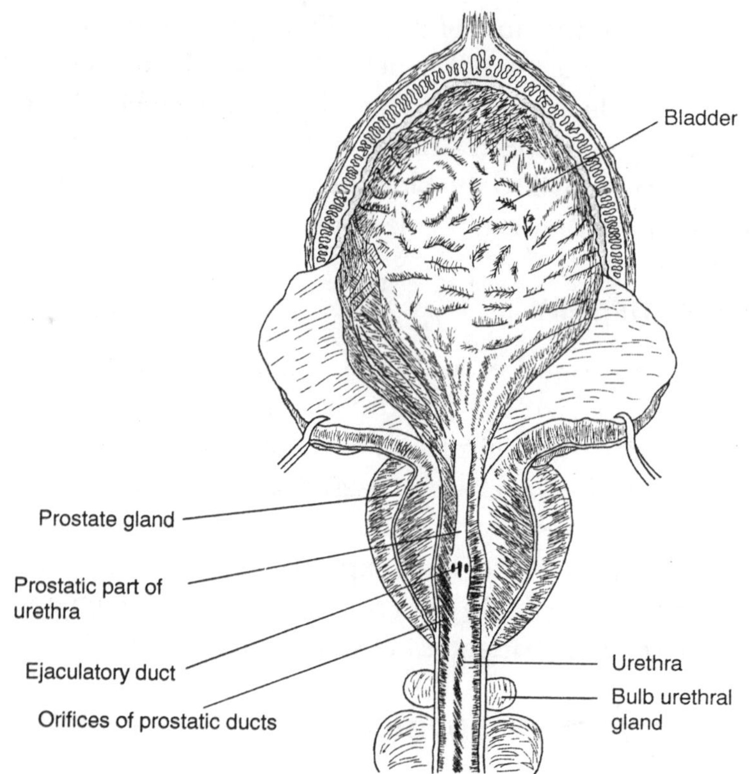

Fig. 5. Transverse Section of the Bladder and Part of the Urethre

prostatectomy. The patients who cannot be operated upon immediately due to other health problems are given preliminary drainage by inserting an urethral catheter followed within 8 to 10 days by prostatectomy. Suprapubic cystostomy is only reserved for very poor risk patients. Preliminary drainage by indwelling urethral catheter has greater acceptance in patients. It permits congestion of the prostate and bladder to subside. In the recess between this stage and the operation, surgeon can do all the necessary investigations. This recess will improve the condition of the patient as well. In the mean time, main emphasis is to lower the blood urea level of the patient. Antibiotic cover given with the operation gives adequate protection against infections.

Types of prostatectomy

There are **four major types of prostatectomy** that are commonly practised.

1. **Supra-pubic prostatectomy**: In this type of operation, the prostate is approached through the bladder. This type of operation has a scientific basis that there is a plane of cleavage between the adenomatous part of the gland and the false capsule composed of compressed normal prostate. It is through this plane of cleavage that the gland is enucleated leaving behind the false capsule, which contracts and forms a scaffold on which the new prostatic urethra is regenerated. The epithelial lining of this regenerated urethra originates from the mucosa above and below.
2. **Retro-pubic prostatectomy:** In this type of operation, the prostate is approached through the retro-pubic space in front of the bladder instead of going via the bladder as is done in supra-pubic prostatectomy.
3. **Transurethral prostatectomy:** When the patient has urinary obstruction and there is no gross enlargement of the prostate gland, particularly of the lateral lobes, this route is adopted for operation. This operation is ideal for small fibrous prostate, middle lobe

enlargement, small adenomatous prostate and carcinoma of the prostate. The resection is done under direct vision either by means of a wire loop diathermy or by a circular punch. Transurethral prostatectomy is a job requiring precision and only specialists can do it. General surgeons do not venture to perform this type of an operation.

4. **Perineal prostatectomy:** As the name indicates, perineal is related to the region of perineum and hence the approach is through urethra by passing a metal bougie and incision is made in front of the anus. This means the surgeon is approaching the prostate body directly. This type of operation is not popular in India.

Post Operative Complications of Prostatectomy

1. Bleeding or **Hemorrhage** is the most serious and important complication following prostatectomy. Clot retention may result from blockage of the catheter or the drainage tube by a blood clot. Continuous bladder wash and instillation of citrate solution helps prevent this complication.
2. A small **infection** after the operation is unavoidable due to the presence of large raw surface in the prostatic bed. Serious degree of sepsis is uncommon unless the bladder was previously infected.
3. **Epididymitis** is another complication. Some surgeons prefer to perform bilateral division of the vas deferens as a routine procedure before prostatectomy to avoid this complication.

4. **Cardiac and respiratory complications**: These complications are likely to occur in early postoperative period because the patients are aged. To avoid these complications, doctors check the condition of cardiac and respiratory organs in the preoperative investigations.

5. **Renal failure:** The surgeon has to correctly ascertain the renal function status before conducting prostatectomy. Prostatectomy is not a minor operation and if the kidneys are not functioning properly due to backpressure, they are likely to fail after the operation. Infusion of fluid should be given very cautiously, since in renal failure excessive fluid intake will aggravate the condition.

6. **Stricture of the bladder neck**: It is likely that a shelf of tissue remains after the removal of prostatic adenoma. This takes part in the generalized contraction of the prostatic bed and causes late stricture formation. Trigonectomy is done to prevent this complication. [Operation of Trigone. Trigone is a triangular area at the base of the bladder between the two ureteral orfices above and laterally and internal urethral orifices below and centrally.]

7. **Osteitis pubis** [Osteitis is the inflammation of whole thickness of the bone including marrow and cortex.]: This postoperative complication arises due to the spread of infection from the retropubic space. When the bony changes have already taken place (common in old persons), the posterior surface of the symphysis pubis is incised and the necrotic cartilage and bone are curetted out.

WHEN IS THERE A NEED FOR OPERATION?

After the doctor conducts rectal examination and the patient undergoes various specific tests like ultrasound, stool, blood and urine examination etc., and prostate enlargement is declared, the patient is eager to know whether he needs an operation of the prostate or not?

- It must be noted that the frequency of urine alone is never an indication for removing the prostate (prostatectomy). Natural progression of benign prostatic enlargement is variable and rarely gets worse even after ten years of passing first, second and third stages as described above. A patient with symptoms of frequent urination for nine years is unlikely to get more symptoms while a similar degree of symptoms reached in three years is a greater indication for surgery.
- Increasing difficulty in micturition with considerable frequency of urine both during day and night, delay in starting urine and a poor stream are the usual symptoms for which prostatectomy is mostly needed.
- Those who are physically fit, can fight the infection of surgical instruments (if any) and have resistance power to recoup health after the operation and are not above eighty years of age are the ideal candidates for surgery.
- Residual urine of 200 cc or more, a raised blood urea, hydroureter or hydronephrosis demonstrated on

urography and uraemic manifestations warrant a need for operation.

- Acute retention of urine, which is not relieved by passing a catheter and emptying the bladder, also calls for an operation.
- Patients who have complications like stone, infection and diverticulum formation need operation.
- Patients who have hemorrhage or venous bleeding from a ruptured vein overlying the prostate, which does not stop with catheter drainage, need immediate operation.
- Permanent installation of a catheter, be it urethral or suprapubic is a rarity and hence prostatectomy or more correctly the removal of the adenomatous (benign cyst) hyperplasia (excessive fluid contents), by one of the four routes, is required.

■

SECTION - III

PROSTATITIS, TUBERCULOUS PROSTATE AND PROSTATIC CALCULI

PROSTATITIS

Prostatitis is the inflammation of the prostate gland mainly due to bacterial spread from urethra. Presence of urinary catheterization may also lead to it. Prostatitis causes pain while passing urine and the frequency also increases. It may even cause fever and discharge of pus. Through rectal examination one can palpate an enlarged prostate. Antibiotics help to clear up the infection. In certain cases, transuretheral prostectomy can be done.

In both acute and chronic prostatitis, it is the seminal vesicles that are usually infected. In some cases, the prostatic urethra is also involved and there is triad of pathological condition. Infection of any one of the structures viz. posterior urethra, prostate and seminal vesicles can occur.

ACUTE PROSTATITIS

ETIOLOGY

In most of the cases of acute prostatitis, the organism responsible is E. Coli. Before the advent of modern research the organism most commonly implicated was Neisseria gonorrheae. The others are Staphylococci and Streptococci. The infection is hematogenous and it may originate from a distant organ, e.g. infected tonsils, carious teeth, furunculosis and diverticulitis. In a few cases, the infection originates from the urethra in ascending fashion or from the kidneys and bladder in the descending order. Acute prostatitis normally results from local extension of an inflammatory process in the urethra or bladder. It may also be due to urethral catheterization. The process of inflammation may involve the entire organ or entail only localized abscesses.

SYMPTOMS, CLINICAL FEATURES

The infection in the prostate is mostly hematological borne and the general manifestations are more prominent than the local. The man suffering from prostatitis has pain all over the body, shivers, feels sick and has backache. There may be fever up to 102° F. All the symptoms resemble influenza. Dysuria is also a common feature. If urine is checked in the first glass, threads are seen. Perineal heaviness, rectal irritation and pain on defecation can also be the associated manifestations. Sitting is very uncomfortable for the patient. Some people also complain of urethral discharge but it is very rare. If the infection spreads up to the bladder, the frequency of urine is more. In case a rectal examination is done, it would reveal a tender prostate and its one lobe is more swollen than the other one. The seminal vesicles may be involved.

PATHOLOGY

When histologic (microscopic study of the structure and function of tissues) examination is done, it reveals neutrophilic (growing optimally in the neutral range of external pH) infiltration of both the stroma (space and aqueous solution enclosed within the inner membrane of a chloroplast) and the glands.

CAUTION AND TREATMENT

One has to seek treatment for this infection. If not treated in time, recurrent attacks follow with severe symptoms. The infection may spread to the epididymes and testes. Urine test will reveal the infection and the patient should be advised to take rest for at least ten days and avoid alcohol. No sexual acts should be undertaken. Normally, antibiotics are prescribed for treatment.

CHRONIC PROSTATITIS

ETIOLOGY AND PATHOGENESIS

When acute prostatitis is not treated in time, it may become chronic. Chronic prostatitis is always a sequel of acute. It is clinically more significant than acute prostatitis due to its high rate of recurrence. In most of the cases, it is a common cause of relapsing urinary tract infection in men. It is difficult to find the organism responsible for it but pus is present in the prostatic secretions. The predominant organism responsible for the infection is E.Coli, Staphylococci, and diptheroids in the order explained. Smears show bacteria in about forty percent of patients and cultures are positive in about seventy percent of the cases.

Both bacterial and nonbacterial conditions exist in chronic prostatitis. Bacterial prostatitis occurs insidiously and not as a consequence of acute prostatits. However, the causative organisms are the same as that for acute prostatitis. Bacterial prostatitis occurs before U.T.I. manifests its symptoms. On the other hand, non-bacterial prostatitis is supposed to have a viral origin. It does not occur before U.T.I. as in the case of bacterial variety. The lumina of the ducts get blocked with epithelial debris and pus. Naturally, the prostate gets enlarged and tender. In the later stage, fibrosis occurs and the prostate becomes smaller and harder.

CLINICAL FEATURES

- The symptoms and clinical features of chronic prostatitis have great variations. It mainly occurs with older men.
- The clinical manifestations are similar for both bacterial and nonbacterial forms of the condition.

- Chronic prostatitis can result in dysuria, urinary frequency and urgency, prostate enlargement and tenderness, although it often may be asymptomatic.
- Acute or mildly acute epididymitis rarely occurs unless prostatitis exists. If it occurs, it is not tuberculous.
- It may cause chronic posterior urethritis and certain tests are needed to confirm it.
- There is dull pain in the rectum and perineum. If the patient sits on a hard surface or chair, the pain aggravates.
- The pain is also experienced in the lower back and may extend towards legs. Such a pain is normally considered as lumbago but it may not be same because it is related to rectum and the perineum. Those who undergo orthopedic or physiotherapy treatment are not much benefited in their lumbago.
- All symptoms that coincide with arthritis, neuritis or even with conjunctivitis are not to be related with symptoms of prostatitis unless formation of pus is present.
- There are recurring attacks of mild fever that lasts for two to three days and is accompanied by malaise.
- Premature ejaculation, prostatorrhea and impotence are the conditions that are generally associated with chronic prostatits.

PATHOLOGY

On histology, it is found that chronic prostatitis is the result of an inflammatory reaction with prominent aggregation [Aggregation of lymphocytes that are non-specific should not be taken as chronic prostatitis because these are due to ageing. Of course, if inflammatory cells exist, the condition should be taken as stated above.] of numerous lymphocytes, plasma cells, macrophages and neutrophils within the glandular acini (type of tumor or cell) and fibrotic stroma. There is large laminated calcification (**Corpora amylacea**) limited within the glands.

DIAGNOSIS

Examination of rectum does not confirm the diagnosis. When the organ is felt soft, it is considered abnormal. When the organ is felt smaller and harder, even then it is abnormal. Usually in mild chronic cases, no change in the organ can be detected. Actual reliability or confirmation of prostatitis is done by pathological examination of the prostatic fluid.

Examination of the prostatic fluid confirms the diagnosis. This fluid can be obtained by massaging the prostate. The normal prostatic fluid is a little opalescent (pertaining to an opal) and viscid (sticky). A stained specimen shows many pus cells and sometimes bacteria.

If urethroscopy is done, it would reveal inflammation of the prostatic urethra and one can see the pus exuding from the prostatic ducts. The verumontanum (Colliculus seminalis) is likely to be enlarged.

FIRST AID FOR URINE PROBLEMS AND PROSTATITIS

[It is better if you consult a naturopath for further guidance in this respect.]

- If there is **burning sensation while passing urine** take fresh juice of **Coriander** (an aromatic plant with seeds and leaves used for flavoring). In Hindi, it is called 'Dhania'. Coriander is a natural diuretic. Prepare tea from the seeds and pour hot water over the strainer in the water to make an infusion. The tea makes the urine more alkaline. There is another method of taking coriander to treat burning of urine and infection of prostate. Soak about 15 grams of coriander seeds in water overnight. In the morning, grind the seeds to a paste, add a cup of water and then filter it through a cloth. Add some ground 'Mishri' (Hindi) to this and drink it in the morning. Repeat for two days.
- Taking five leaves of **Basil ('Tulsi'in Hindi)** everyday is a great preventive for any urine infection like burning in urine and retention of urine. If there is burning sensation in urine, take 20 leaves of 'Tulsi' and swallow them with water after some chewing for sometime between tongue and palate. Tulsi should not be chewed with teeth.
- If there is **loss of control over the flow of urine** and it spurts involuntarily, take **Nutmeg** duly grinded with water. It is a hard, fragrant tropical seed which is grounded or grated as a spice. In Hindi, it is called 'Jaiphal'.
- If there is **pain while urinating** and you have been diagnosed for prostatitis, along with medicines

prescribed, you can take milk with **Turmeric powder**. In a glass of warm milk, add half a teaspoonful of turmeric powder, dissolve it and drink it at breakfast.

- In Prostatitis, fresh gel of **Aloe vera** is useful. This is available in the market in liquid packs under the name of 'Kumari Saar'. One tablespoonful of Aloe vera, three times a day is useful. It is anti-inflammatory, a blood purifier and a coolant for the body. In almost every disease, Aloe Vera can be taken.
- If you feel very much **weak and drained because of urine problems**; scanty, dribbling or frequent urine, take a cup of milk in the morning and evening. This milk should be heated in a **silver vessel**, allowed to get lukewarm and then taken.
- Taking Ginger can treat **pain during urination and haematuria**. Take **dry ginger** ('Saunth' in Hindi), grind it and filter the powder through a cloth. Mix some ground 'Mishri' in it. Half a teaspoonful of this mixture is to be put in one cup of milk and taken three times a day.

GRANULOMATOUS PROSTATITIS

"Granulomatous" strictly means *containing form of granules with inflammation*. It is of two types:

The first type is **nonspecific granulomas** (a circumscribed mass or nodule consisting mainly of histiocytes) that are secondary to either acute prostatitis or chronic prostatitis. The cause has been attributed to retention of prostatic secretions. Histological examination reveals inflammatory cells with well circumscribed granulomas of epithelial giant cells with traces of eosinophils.

The second type is **tuberculosis of the prostate gland.** It usually follows tuberculosis of the genitourinary tract. This subject is taken up in detail below.

TUBERCULOSIS OF THE PROSTATE

Tuberculosis of the prostate and seminal vesicles co-exists with renal tuberculosis in at least sixty percent of the cases. In half of such cases, there is history of pulmonary tuberculosis within five years of the onset of genital tuberculosis.

Tuberculosis of prostate is not very common. Tuberculosis of seminal vesicles, one or both is much more common. When examining a patient with chronic tuberculous epididymitis, there is no symptom referred to internal genitalia. It is on examining rectum that one finds vesicles affected. It may be nodular and tender. In the process of time, tuberculous seminal vesiculitis may further lead to congestion and edema of the base of the bladder, the latter to basal cystitis.

In case of tuberculosis of prostate, the rectal examination would reveal one or more well-defined nodules near the upper or lower border of one or both the lateral lobes. In some cases, a large single mass is felt occupying a near central position. Nodules in the prostate do not have the stony hardness that is found in carcinoma of prostate.

SYMPTOMS

- As a matter of rule, a urethral discharge is the first symptom of tuberculosis of prostate. In the event of this symptom, differential diagnosis has to be made for gonorrhea and a bacterial urethritis totally depending upon bacteriological findings. Prostate, in the first stage of tuberculosis is generally felt normal.
- In about twenty five percent of the cases, there are painful, blood stained ejaculations.
- There is mild pain in the perineum.
- There is reduction of fertility for those who have tuberculous prostatitis or even bilateral seminal vesiculitis. Eighty percent of cases are sterile. A male is always worried about fertility and tuberculous prostato-vesiculitis can be diagnosed by examining culture of semen.
- When the tuberculosis lingers for some time without treatment, the posterior urethra gets involved either via direct extention from the prostate or by the discharge of a prostatic abscess. In such a case, the micturition is painful and sometimes hematuria also occurs.

INVESTIGATIONS

Radiography

In radiography, some areas of calcification in the prostate and/or the seminal vesicles can be seen. If the area of calcification is large and scattered, it is a sign of tuberculosis rather than endogenous prostatic calculi.

Bacterial examination

Bacteriological examination of the seminal fluid gives positive culture for tubercle bacilli in most cases of tuberculous prostate.

Posterior urethrography

Posterior urethrography generally reveals one or more dilated prostatic ducts. Typically they are multiple and gaping. If the ducts are dilated, it is indicative of chronic prostatitis. Dilated prostatic ducts are not specific for tuberculosis. On the other hand, if the ducts are dilated and in addition, there is finding of tubercle bacilli in the ejaculate (semen), confirms the diagnosis of tuberculosis.

CALCULI OF PROSTATE

Calculi as we know are formations of stones. Prostatic calculi are of two kinds. One is endogenous and the other is exogenous.

Exogenous calculi [Exogenous means produced from outside the organism.] are comparatively rare. They are mostly urinary calculus, which get arrested in the prostatic urethra. As a matter of rule, calculi occur less frequently in the urethra than in any other part of the urinary tract. A urethral calculus can arise primarily in the urethra behind a stricture or in an infected urethral diverticulum. There is very little scope for a calculus that has migrated from the ureter to large in the prostatic bulbous or penile portions of the urethra. **Migratory calculi can be arrested in the urethra of children below the age of two years because they have a large vesicle neck.**

Endogenous [Endogenous is produced from within, internal, occurring or controlled from within the organism.] prostatic calculi are mostly composed of calcium phosphate and organic material. Most of the cases of endogenous calculi asymptomatic and are discovered on radiography of pelvis when the patient is getting prostatectomy done. The symptoms if present, vary in severity and are at first those of chronic prostatitis or of prostatic obstruction.

If rectal examination is done, the calculus is difficult to differentiate from carcinoma of prostate. On the X-Ray film, the stones appear in the shape of horseshoe or a circle.

Endogenous calculi generally do not warrant the need for doctor's consultation because they do not manifest any exclusive symptoms and also do not create problems. When symptoms like retention of urine, frequent urination, pain in the region etc. occur, then prostatitis is the first presumptive diagnosis and if calculi is associated with it as confirmed by various tests, prostatectomy is undertaken.

■

SECTION - IV

CANCER OF PROSTATE GLAND

CANCER

The name of disease **prostatic cancer** is a terror for the patient and his relatives/friends. Somehow cancer has become a synonymous of death. The terror is more than the disease. It is being cured successfully in certain conditions.

There is a dogmatic understanding among public that cancer is incurable. This is not true. The medical world has evidence that it can be cured. **'Early diagnosis, Better prognosis'** stands true for cancer. Prime causation that produces or promotes cancer is not known but there are reasons to believe that one of the causes explained here below could be the culprit to trigger cancer.

POSSIBLE CAUSATIVE FACTORS OF CANCER

- Deficiency of potassium.
- Excessive consumption of salted food and use of bicarbonate of soda in preparation of certain foods.

- Living in polluted atmosphere and hence less of oxygen intake.
- Excessive/indiscreet use of orthodox toxic drugs that have side effects.
- Anger, worry, brooding and getting highly emotional on petty matters.
- Chronic constipation.
- Inhaling some poisonous fumes, exposure to X-rays, radioactive rays, contact with irritating substances and chemicals.
- Vaccination, injuries, chewing tobacco and alcoholism.
- Tattoo on the skin.
- Excessive use of alcohol, smoking, chewing tobacco and other stimulating offences.
- Frequent pregnancies.
- Wounds, injuries, animal/insect bites, complicated bone fractures etc.
- Frequent attacks of Malaria and its wrong medication.
- Surgical incisions.

Let us see what research scholars have said about cancer.

- **Cancer can be cured by medicines and not by surgery**, say Dr. Deelman and Dr. Murphy after they conducted number of experiments. (Chapter nine of the book, 'Cancer, the surgeon and researcher' by Ellis Barker). Dr. Deelman further says that **Cancerous growth is**

excited by surgical incisions and this he proved on rats.

- According to another study, **Cancer is not a local irritation but a blood condition**, which causes an outbreak in one or another weakened spot. (Journal of Experimental Medicine, U.S.A.-1925)
- **Cancer is not infectious** and even if a healthy person is transfused blood of a person suffering from cancer, it would have no effect. (please refer 'Victory Over Cancer' by Cyril Scott.)

Doctor Gamer, Jordan and Haraknes wrote a letter the British Medical Journal in 1938 stating that cancer is the disease of civilization. It is due to conventionalism and bad eating habits of civilization and deviation from natural and normal state of health of the alimentary tract. In villages, where the natives have not lost touch with the first principle of feeding and have no constipation due to proper food intake, there is no cancer. Whether this statement is true or not cannot be said but one **aspect of cancer is clear that it is a product of going away from natural foods and resorting to junk food in tins, foils etc. with use of so called 'permitted' colors and artificial scents.** Places where such types of food called 'fast food' have not reached, are generally free of cancer.

Cancer by heredity has been ruled out according to a recent study and it can be thought of as a constitutional disease. But according to a famous homeopath, **John H. Clarke, MD**. 'Cancer is a complex disease and the formation of tumor may be regarded as the final chapter of the series. Heredity plays an important part; contagion plays a, perhaps, sometimes less important part; and other factors sometimes play an all important part quite independently, as it seems, of the other two. Blood poisoning of many kinds may be determining factor in the causation of cancer. (Reference from 'Cure of Tumours by Medicines,' B. Jain Publishers, page 17). Further he adds, that there is close alliance between the tubercular and cancerous diatheses. In families with strong tubercular taint, some develop tuberculosis while others develop cancer. Gout is a factor of no less importance than either of the other two."(Page 165).

FEAR OF CANCER IN PROSTATE

Whenever there is problem in urination in old age, people go to the doctor for consultation and medication. A friend of mine was not afraid of drugs and treatment when doctors told him that he had enlarged prostate. His fear was cancer of prostate although tests were not done to trace cancer. It so happened that after his PSA was taken, it turned out to be positive. It is a test to know whether the organ is benign or cancerous. He was promptly advised surgery but his relatives and friends did not approve of it because he was seventy-six years old. At this age when cancer is diagnosed, people in general do not go in for operations. His health otherwise was good. He was monetarily stable and independent of any liabilities. The doctor felt that his operation if undertaken would help him live more. My friend consulted another three doctors to take their opinion. Two of them advised prostatectomy but one of them told him to postpone the surgery and carry on with life with some changes in diet and resorting to 'Yoga'. Swami Ramdev of Haridwar is in news now a days and this had probably impressed the doctor. There was confusion for my friend now. Three doctors were in favour of the operation and one was against it.

What do you think, this old man should do? The opinions may vary but one thing is sure that prostate cancer did not develop overnight. It had taken tens of years to develop and he was not aware of it till his symptoms like retention of urine, dribbling and frequency etc. started. So far he was living with cancer of prostate, of course not knowing it. Ignorance is really bliss in such cases. Once he knew that he suffered from cancer, not only he but also his kith and kin were fearfully worried. This man is a retired government officer and his son is a homeopathic doctor. I knew this man casually but his son is well known to me. I had met him in one of the seminars. His son sought my advice on the condition of his father. I told him not to resort to operation and that he should try homeopathic medicines.

In the field of medicine, we, the doctors, have a tragic shortcoming at our own homes. We are not considered doctors for our family members. Let a doctor be a reputed and well known doctor for the public but for family members, there is no belief in his/her treatment. *"Ghar ka Jogi jogra, Bahar ka jogi sidh'* is a saying in Hindi. It means that a saint is real saint for outsiders but not for his family.

This is what had happened at the home of this young doctor whose father had prostate cancer. He had already suggested his father not to go for operation and take homeopathic medicines but his father had no belief in homeopathic medicines. On his request, I paid a visit to his home and discussed with his father about the operation and cancer of prostate. After a thoughtful consideration, he agreed to postpone the operation and take homeopathic medicines. We suggested a change in his diet routine and work. He was also advised some 'yoga' exercises. Initially he was given *Cantharis* 30 since he was having burning in urine. After three days, when burning of urine subsided, *Sabal serrulata* Q was started. He has been taking only five drops of this medicine daily for twenty five days in a month since four years and not having any prostate problem. I had told the patient to get the prostate checked but now he was not ready. ' Let it be there, I have been living with it for decades, so be it there. I am feeling fine and have no problem. Cancer has befriended me', used to be his reply. It is certain that fear or phobia of cancer is more dangerous than actual cancer. In this case, microscopic malignancy appears to have been eradicated and the size of prostate reduced considerably otherwise the patient would have made complaints in his urination act. He is now nearing eighty and has no urine problem. **The will to live works more than the fear of dying.** This 'will' to live comes only on initiation from well-wishers, self meditation and conducting 'yoga'. I do not know whether it was his 'will to live', homeopathic medicines or regular 'Yoga' that cured him.

Many doctors in the western countries believe that enlargement of prostate is linked with cancer of prostate. This is the reason why surgeons in India also advice prostatectomy even when they find benign prostate hypertrophy. According to an estimate, over four lakh cases in **USA are diagnosed as prostate cancer and over three lakh persons die of cancer of prostate every year.** Prostatic problems have reached epidemic proportions. According to the, statement published by a drug company of USA, if someone has an enlarged prostate, the risk of developing cancer is more. This is the reason that after 65 years of age, prostatectomy is the second most common surgery performed on men in USA. TURP (transurethral resection of prostate) is a very common surgery there and is known as *'roto-rooter job'*. BHP is a well known disease and you will be surprised that people have established Prostate Cancer Research Institute in USA like that of Diabetic, Cancer and Thyroid institutes.

It has been established that Prostate is most susceptible to cancer than any other human organ in the body. In USA, lung cancer claims more lives but cancer of prostate is not far behind. It rates as the second most lethal male cancer. By the age of 65 years, almost two out of three persons may have slight cancer or so called microscopic cancer in their prostates although the symptoms are existent.

The most astonishing fact about cancer (not only of prostate) is that the persons having cancer are unaware of its presence for a number of years. Prostate cancer also grows slowly. It takes about twenty to thirty years for the prostate to grow large enough for detection by the modern tests available for the purpose. There are no serious problems when the cancer grows. **People die of other associated problems like heart disease and kidney failure and not from prostate cancer**. By the time cancer of prostate reaches an explosive stage, the person dies either of natural ageing or of cardiac or diabetic problems. The reason of prostate cancer is still unknown but some research scholars say that excess fat raises level of testosterone (a male hormone) and it promotes cancer growth. Low fat intake can, therefore, half the progression of tiny malignant tumors or treated their growth so that they are not life threatening. Best is to avoid fat after the age of fifty. Everybody knows it but still the "good food greed" of old men exists, at least in India.

It is not known whether enlargement of prostate affects first or cancer of prostate starts before the enlargement of prostate. Enlargement of prostate to the extent of producing symptoms take tens of years and so does the growth of cancer.

CANCER PHOBIA

Now I come to cancer phobia. Cancer has spread to such an extent that people not suffering from cancer also fear that its presence. Slight disorders like continued coryza, cough, ulcers in mouth, infection in urine etc., make them think of cancer first. This is cancer phobia. Recently, AIDS has taken over from cancer and people think of it also.

Cancer has no link with heredity but still this cancer phobia prevails in persons whose kith and kin had history of cancer. It is also in persons who have read more about cancer and seen cancer deaths in neighborhood. Seeing cancer death in the near relatives or neighborhood is still very fearful. One sees the person hale and hearty and suddenly he or she goes on getting weak day by day. After the treatment like chemotherapy starts, one sees the person losing his or her hair. And one day he or she dies. Seeing such a horrible death makes the person sad and depressed. If this fear psychosis stimulates one's brain to the extent of constant worry and tension, the first stage of cancer may erupt if one is under polluted atmosphere and has wrong eating habits. Those who are suffering this sort of phobia should consult the doctor. If such people hesitate to go to doctor, the relatives should press them to get examined.

DIFFERENCE BETWEEN CANCER AND BENIGN TUMOURS?

Every one knows the name of this disease and its consequences but few persons actually know its meaning, growth and outcome. Cancer is rapid and abnormal cellular proliferation, a new growth of cells. Cancer growth is characterized by certain definite peculiarities of metabolism, structure and association. Cancer cell has characteristics that make it different from other types of cells. This obvious new growth in the body is known as 'Neoplasm'. It means progressive, parasitic and often disruptive proliferation. This growth goes on spreading at the expense of other normal cells of the organism at slow or rapid rate. 'Neoplasm' is also known as tumor that has features of local swelling and enlargement. It is mostly hard and does not yield to pressure. It does not pit and is generally localized whereas swelling edema pits on pressure and covers large area of skin. If it is not tumor, it may be termed as a cyst. Cyst is filled with fluid and it yields to pressure. 'Neoplasm' is of two types: Benign and Malignant.

BENIGN TUMOUR

Benign tumors do not grow rapidly and remain localized, encapsulated and have no tendency to infiltrate. They generally do not affect their neighboring organs. Their intention is to disorganize the tissues. They spread locally and there is no dissemination to other parts of the body by metastasis and they do not recur after excision. Benign tumor cells are almost similar to the tissues and of uniform size and shape with nuclei resembling mature cell type nuclei, of normal color stain with few and well formed blood vessels. The stroma is arranged in big bands and hemorrhages and ulcerations do not occur.

MALIGNANT TUMOR

Malignant or cancerous tumors grow rapidly and they do not have a tendency for encapsulation. They remain localized but infiltrate the neighboring tissues. They are harmful to the host as they swallow the nourishment of the host and produce toxic products leading to anemia, wasting, cachexia and finally death. They disorganize the tissues and form open ulcers. They spread by @ metastasis [Metastasis is one of the most characteristic feature of malignant tumors and it is the actual ability to spread.] and disseminate to lymphatics, blood vessels and nerves. If they are cut, they reoccur after excision where from hemorrhage and ulcer formation is common. Their cells are variable in shape and size and exhibit typical mitotic figures and multiple nuclei having hyper chromatic stain. Most of the blood vessels are ill formed and lined by malignant cells. The stroma [Stroma is the space and aqueous solution enclosed within the inner membrane of a chloroplast.] is fine and reticulate.

All tumors have two basic ingredients, proliferating neoplastic cells that consists of the parenchyma of the tumor and supportive stroma made of connective tissues and blood vessels. We shall not go into further details of cancerous tumors or growth. We can brief now by stating that 'Cancer spreads crab-like extensions in the surrounding tissue that make localized enucleating (surgically removing) of malignancy extremely difficult'. Cancer tumors are spreading and we have very limited means to treat them. According to a survey in 1997, every year five lakh people die of cancer in India.

CONDITION IN BENIGN AND MALIGNANT TUMORS

Condition	Benign	Malignant
Bleeding	Non-bleeding	Excessive, prostate, uterus, neck and lungs
Growth rate	Very slow	Very fast
Cells longevity	Normal	Abnormal
Capsule	A round capsule around tumor	No capsule, except in kidney tumors
Ulceration	No	Present
Regrowth	No	Yes
Size of tumor	Usually small	Usually large
Pain	Absent or rare	Mostly painful
Cell multiplication rate	Slow	Very fast
Cell maturation	Good	Cells often immature
Cell function	Restored	Lost
Tissue architecture	Maintained	Lost
Superadded infection	Absent	Common
Prognosis	Good	Mostly poor

CARCINOMA OF THE PROSTATE

[We have used the word carcinoma to depict cancer. A malignant tumor arising from the epithelial tissue is called '**carcinoma**' and a malignant tumor arising out of connective tissue is known as '**sarcoma**'. Generally, benign tumor is designated by attaching the suffix '**oma**' to the cell type from which it arises. A benign tumor arising from fibrous tissue is called '**fibroma**'. A cartilaginous tumor is called 'chondroma' and an epithelial benign tumor arising out of a gland is called '**adenoma**'. **Since this is a basic book for knowledge sake, please take cancer and carcinoma as similar terms although they are different in case of prostate gland.**]

It is a real puzzle to diagnose the case of cancer of prostate in the early stage and it is still difficult to diagnose the case before the neoplasm has spread beyond the anatomical capsule of the prostate. It also happens that cancer was not suspected before enucleation (cutting process of nerves etc. in operation) was undertaken with the diagnosis that it was a case of benign hypertrophy of the prostate. At the time of enucleation, the gland appears to be fixed poteriorly and enucleation then becomes difficult. It is, therefore, essential to make a definite diagnosis of cancer through histopathological tests.

Skin, lungs, breast and pancreas are the most common parts of the body to develop cancer. It can also develop in bone marrow, lymphatic system and bones. Other parts of body may have cancer but they are not much prone to it. **Prostate gland** is one of them which is supposed to be free of cancer provided some diet measures are taken in time when the man is in his fifties. The growth of cancer begins when the oncogens in a cell or cells are transformed by agents known as *carcinogens.* Years may pass before the growth of cells cause symptoms. Even during occult phase, metastasis may develop in lungs, liver, bones and brain. In most cases, confirmation of cancer is done by biopsy.

Carcinoma of the prostate is a common malignant condition in men over the age of fifty years or so. About thirty percent of cases of prostatic obstruction turn out to be due to carcinoma. The cases of cancer of prostate are on the increase in India due to longevity in old men. Prostate cancer normally occurs and originates in the external group of glands. Hence, prostatectomy for benign enlargement of the gland confers little protection from the subsequent development of carcinoma.

The type of **carcinoma is latent** in many cases. At the beginning we have stated that if men lived more than seventy-five years of age, every man will have cancerous prostate but in most of the cases, degree of prostatic cancer is not much. Many of these neoplasms are tiny and might have remained latent for years, had they not been investigated by test. It, therefore, appears that a seedling carcinoma is often present in the prostate of an elderly man awaiting favorable conditions to become active. In USA, it is called microscopic carcinoma and with every enlargement of prostate, it is supposed present in most of cases.

The prostate cancer is spheroidal celled with a degree of tubule formation. The tumor is hence slow in growth. They are graded in two classes: **Anaplastic** and **Adenocarcinoma**. Anaplastic type is more malignant and manifests itself more aggressively than an adeno-carcinoma.

Bone is a common site of distant metastasis of prostate cancer. These metastases are normally osteoblastic, showing areas of increased density on skeletal X-ray. Prostate cancer can involve any portion of the gland but most commonly arises in the periphery. Most prostate cancers are of epithelial origin (adenocarcinomas) and not sarcomas (mesenchymal origin) and such types of cancers are associated with elevated serum levels of prostate specific antigen and prostatic acid phosphatase, not human chorionic gonadotropin. Nearly 75% of prostatic carcinomas are thought to originate in the posterior lobe of the gland.

SPREAD OF CARCINOMA

SPREAD BY LOCAL INVASION

The **spread of carcinoma of prostate** is localized. A growth commencing in the posterior zone of the gland is prevented temporarily from extending backwards by the strong fascia of Denonvilliers (Rectovesical septum).

In the next stage, it starts to grow upwards to involve **the seminal vesicles**. If it grows further upwards and extends, it would obstruct the lower end of **one or both the ureters**, the latter terminating in anuria.

Further in the next stage, carcinoma commencing in a lateral lobe would involve the **prostatic urethra** early and in very advanced stage, the base of bladder is also invaded by cancer. It is observed that rectum is involved very occasionally by the infiltration causing stricture of the rectal wall. **The mucosa does not ulcerate unless traumatized for e.g. by transrectal biopsy**.

BY BLOOD STREAM

Spread of cancer by blood occurs particularly to bones. Prostate is the most common site of origin for skeletal metastases, being followed in turn by breasts, kidneys, the bronchial tree and the thyroid gland. The pelvic bones and lower lumbar vertebrae are particularly affected. The frequent proximity of skeletal metastases to the primary growth is because of reversed flow from the vesicle venous plexus to the emissary veins of the pelvic bones especially during the act of coughing, sneezing etc.

SPREAD BY LYMPH

Lymphatic spread of carcinoma is through lymphatic vessels passing along the sides of the rectum to the lymph nodes along the internal iliac vein and in the hollow of the sacrum. It also spreads via lymphatics to the seminal vesicles and follow the vas deferens for a short distance to drain into the external iliac lymph nodes. The retroperitoneal lymph nodes and then the mediastinal nodes and occasionally the supraclavicuar lymph nodes also get involved through either of the above mentioned routes.

PATHOLOGY

Prostatic carcinomas characteristically appear as nodular, ill-defined areas of stone hard consistency from gray- white to yellow.

In **histologic appearance**, most of prostatic carcinomas are adenocarcinomas having glandular structure. One can see two types of cells; clear cells and dark spindle cells.

Clear cells have abundant foamy cytoplasm and **dark spindle cells** have condensed cytoplasm. It is also observed that normal lobular structure is destroyed due to irregular growth of the malignant acini (tumor or cell). Perineural invasion is a common finding.

Grading prostate cancer depends upon the degree of glandular differentiation and the pattern of growth in relation to the stroma.

PREDISPOSING FACTORS

There is a clear association of prostate cancer with old age mostly over fifty years and one cannot forget its connection with racial backgrounds. It has a high prevalence in blacks as compared to Asians. It is also established that environmental influence also plays a part in initiating cancer as is found in persons who are exposed to cadmium or catch viral infections in their professional chores.

CLINICAL FEATURES

- It is difficult to define the symptoms of cancer of prostate because they are variable and can only be diagnosed by some tests. Most of the people do not undergo pathological tests and hence the detection of cancer is not made in time.
- So far study of cancer of prostate suggests that carcinoma of the prostate occurs in older men at an early age than the age by which they attain benign enlargement of prostate. This means that cancer of prostate starts earlier than the benign enlargement. **After the enlargement has occurred in prostate, the chances of carcinoma are there but they are less.**
- The very first symptom of cancer of prostate is acute or chronic retention of urine.
- The symptoms and signs of benign enlargement of prostate and prostate cancer are almost identical.
- The symptoms and signs of benign enlargement of prostate are same as that of to prostate cancer but the history of disease in benign cases is short, say weeks, not months. A hard nodule or increased fixation of the gland favors the diagnosis of carcinoma.
- There is pain in the perineum or suprapubic region besides symptoms of prostatic obstruction in the patient. When rectal examination is done, a possibility of carcinoma is doubted if there is finding of an indurated area in the gland.

- Carcinoma of prostate may arise in any lobe but it generally originates in the posterior lobe, near the outer margins.
- When the urinary symptoms do not exist or they are minimal but there is pain in the back or sciatica is present, it is a doubtful case of cancer. Bilateral sciatica in old persons is most often on account of metastases in the spine from carcinoma of the prostate.
- Microscopic or occult cancer is asymptomatic and urinary symptoms appear only when tumor has already spread. Pain in the region is a late symptom that reflects involvement of capsular periurethral spaces.
- Patients with carcinoma of the prostate may present with acute retention of urine. Relatively sudden attack of dysuria accompanied with very short history of other urinary troubles will give rise to suspicion of cancer. In such a case, rectal examination will confirm the diagnosis.
- Edema of one or both the legs, paraplegia and a spontaneous fracture are occasionally due to metastases from a carcinoma of the prostate. Anemia may also be the presenting symptom.
- Officers working in Insurance companies have a notion that if a man or woman at the age of forty years lose 20% of his or her normal weight, there is danger of cancer and/or consumption or Bright's disease. I do not know whether it is true or not but commercially,

the insurance agents abide by this rule and it must have some background. Who would like to lose money and take risk of insuring such a person?

RECTAL EXAMINATION

Rectal examination would show irregular indurations, characteristically stony hard (a part or the whole of the gland) and a decreased mobility suggests cancer. In some cases, the rectal mucosa is felt 'tethered' (roped or chained) to the back of the prostate by infiltration of the carcinoma. Obliteration of the notch between the seminal vesicles or of the groove between the lateral lobes is suspected as cancer. In addition to this, if the induration extends beyond the lateral limits of the gland causing obliteration of the lateral part or of the membranous urethra, the diagnosis is certain for cancer. Diagnosis of carcinoma of prostate becomes difficult when there are prostatic calculi and calcareous changes secondary to tuberculosis of the seminal vesicles.

DIAGNOSIS

RADIOLOGICAL EXAMINATION (X-RAY)

Radiological examination is done to confirm the diagnosis or exclude the presence of prostatic calculi or pelvic and lumbar skeletal metastases. Osseous metastases from carcinomas of other organs are usually osteolytic producing a rarefied *'moth-eaten'* appearance. Carcinoma in the lower lumbar vertebrae and pelvic bones of the prostate are typically osteoblastic (pertaining to bone forming cells), resulting in increased density of the bones and must be distinguished from Padget's disease of the bone. [Paget disease is a generalized disease of bone due to unknown cause. Males after the age of forty are generally affected. Major development occurs in skull, tibia is bent anteriorly and the femur outward. Enlargement of many other bones occur : oral/jaw bones including pelvic bones. There is no treatment of padget's disease.]

EXAMINATIONS TO FIND OUT METASTASES OF CANCER

[We have used the word 'metastasis' many a times in this book. Metastasis is distant spread of tumor cells anywhere in the body from primary location. This is a very important characteristic of malignant tumor. During metastasis, the tumor cells spread either via the lymphatics or the blood vessels or in some cases via the nerve sheath or other tissue spaces.]

1. Scalene node biopsy

A lymph node is removed from the front of the left scalenus anterior muscle of the neck and biopsy is made of that lymph nose.

2. Bone scanning

Bone scanning is done with radioactive bromine or selenium. The deposits are shown as 'hot spots'.

3. Bone marrow aspiration (sternum or ileum).

This test can find out metastatic carcinoma cells in a high percentage of those cases where radiological examination revealed no evidence of secondary deposits.

This investigation should be made in every case before radical prostatectomy is even considered.

4. Lymphangiography

It is similar to radiography where opaque renal or ureteric calculi are seen. X-ray in this case will show whether there are deposits in the pelvic lymph nodes or any lymphatic obstruction.

5. Serum Acid Phosphtase

Acid phophase is found raised above normal in about forty percent of cases of prostate carcinoma. A reading between 3 to 5 units is suspicious of carcinoma of the prostate whereas a reading above five is diagnostic of carcinoma. The normal reading is one to three King Armstrong unit. If there is extensive bone marrow involvement, very high level up to 100 or more K.A. units are read.

6. Cysto-urethroscopy

This test has already been discussed in BPH chapter under the heading 'Pathological tests' on page 47. When there is a history of hmaturia, this test is essential.

7. Confirmation of the Diagnosis

Examining the histological material from the prostate does confirm of the diagnosis. A true biopsy of the prostatic tissue is obtained with a 'Turkel' needle passed through the perineum into any suspicious area. This open type of biopsy is much in vogue.

8. Transurethral Biopsy

Transurethral resection of prostate has the advantage of removing the obstruction and providing large pieces of tissue. The difficulty is that it may not reach the posterior zone of the prostate and this zone is commonly affected by early carcinoma. It is well known that benign enlargement of prostate and cancer frequently co-exist.

9. Prostate Specific Antigen (PSA) Test

It is a protein developed by the cells of the prostate gland. This test finds out the level of PSA in blood. Generally, PSA level is low in men but in the case of benign or cancerous condition of prostate, PSA level is found increased. PSA level alone does not give sufficient information to confirm benign or cancerous prostate. (PSA level below 4 mg/ml is normal.)

The problem with PSA test is that it cannot distinguish between aggressive tumors and those that would remain slow growing for years leading to over treatment according to opinion of some experts.

TREATMENT IN GENERAL

The conventional treatment is based upon antiandrogenic therapy, which means **orchiectomy and estrogen therapy besides radiotherapy and chemotherapy.**

PROGNOSIS

Tumors, which are well differentiated and have not metastasized are linked with a good five to fifteen years of survival. It is common to see cases when eventually the cancer relapses and spreads to the most frequent sites of metastases. These sites may be regional lymph nodes, bones, lungs, liver and brain. According to some doctors, a man of 65 years and above should not go for orchiectomy, radiotherapy and chemotherapy due to the reason that with cancer, they can survive for more than ten years. This is controversial but many people above sixty-five do not opt for operations.

BODY GIVES A SIGNAL WHEN CANCER ATTACKS

Whatever the case may be, every disease gives signals of its outcome when it attacks the body. Cancer is no exception and it does give symptoms (may be late symptoms) which may be one of the following in males and females:

- Growth of a fibroid, a hard swelling in the breast or any part of the body.
- An injury that is not healing for a long time inspite of treatment.
- Bleeding from the nipples.
- Problems in swallowing simple food.

- Continuous cough and hoarseness or sore throat that is not responding to treatment.
- Change in habits of urination and stool.
- A boil or pimple that does not heal or becomes hard.
- A sudden change in size or color of a long standing wart or corn on the body.
- Bleeding from genitals after coition-male or female.
- Offensive leucorrhea with blood after the age of 45 years..
- Fibroids and/or cysts in uterus, ovaries.
- Stomatitis (mouth ulcers) that do not heal even after medication for a period of more than a month.
- Restart of menses after a menopause.
- Loss of weight and no hunger, continued indigestion. Officers working in Insurance companies have a notion that if a person at the age of forty years loss 20% of his or her normal weight, there is danger of cancer, consumption or Bright disease.

If any one of these above symptoms appear and do not cure in fifteen days or so, better consult a doctor.

TREATMENT OF CANCER OF PROSTATE

Carcinoma of prostate is treated/operated, according to the stage of the disease or the pathological type of tumour.

LATENT CARCINOMA (STAGE I)

The term 'latent' used here signifies that there is no evidence of tumor on clinical examination but cancer is detected histologically in tissues removed from prostatectomy. Investigations show no evidence of metastasis. This term 'latent' should not be confused with 'occult carcinoma'. Occult means that the patient presents with metastasis while the primary tumour remains hidden. It is reasonable to think in case of latent carcinomas that there is no need for treatment of well differentiated local carcinoma, detected in prostatic specimens removed at the operation. In case of more of diffusion and less well-differentiated tumors, repeated examinations should be carried out and active treatment should be undertaken.

CARCINOMA CONFINED TO THE PROSTATE (STAGE II)

In this case, there will be small nodules and a large tumor. They deform the contour of the prostate but are still within the capsule of prostate. These tumors are not common and possibly represent less than five percent of cases presenting with prostatic cancer.

LOCALLY ADVANCED DISEASE (STAGE III)

Many cases, say 30 to 50 % of patients, presenting with prostate cancer have locally extensive disease with no evidence of distant metastasis. Fifty percent of these patients have node metastasis. The results of radical prostatectomy are poor in this group of patients. The capsule appears to provide an effective barrier against the spread of tumor and once this is breached, dissemination of the disease is likely to occur. Under such circumstances, local treatment to the prostate alone will not eliminate the disease. They should be given endocrine therapy.

DISSEMINATED DISEASE (STAGE IV)

In many cases, say 30 to 50 % of patients with prostatic cancer have distant metastases at the time of presentation in surgery. For them hormonal therapy is the best.

■

SECTION - V

CARE AND CURE OF PROSTATE CANCER

We already know that no other human organ is as susceptible to cancer as is the prostate gland. According to a study in USA, two out of every three men at the age of sixty-five in USA have microscopic cancer growth in their prostates.

The care of diseased prostate is needed when it is known that cancer has affected the organ. Besides the care of prostate as explained above, there is lot more required for the care of cancerous prostate.

- There is a belief that **modifying the dietary habits** stall the progress of cancer.
- Go lean on **your fat intake**. Full cream milk, 'Malai', market available and pasteurized cheese and butter should be reduced considerably. Some doctors think that excess of fat intake raises the levels of testosterone, the male sex hormone, which is supposed to promote cancer growth.

- Some doctors are of the opinion that fish if taken in limited quantity; say once or twice in a week is helpful to stall cancer growth. It is seen in a study that people living in coastal area where fish is taken regularly have comparatively less of prostate diseases. Bengalis of eastern India are not much prone to prostate problems as compared to people of northern India.
- It is noted that consumption of **soya** foods (beans, oil and flour) benefits patients of prostate cancer. Men in Japan eat lots of soya food and got benefit from two substances found in soya what lowers the progression of cancer. These two substances are: *genistein* and *genistin* and these reduce the production of testosterone that is believed to aggravate the growth of prostate cancer.
- According to a study undertaken by Harvard School of Public Health, USA, it is said that **lycopene**, an antioxidant compound that gives tomatoes their red color, helps cure cancer.
- **Tomatoes** contain vitamin A, B and C more than oranges and grapes. Even on heating, its vitamins do not get destroyed. Tomatoes have calcium, phosphorus, iron, protein, fat and carbohydrates and give 20 calories of energy. It improves liver functions. If taken early morning, one feels very energetic and passes urine in abundance. A cup of tomato soup everyday helps prevent prostate cancer. It stalls the growth of cancer. Lycopene found in tomatoes is also found in pink grapefruit and watermelon but not much

research has been done on these fruits. Tomato is one of the best vegetables that can be taken raw or cooked.

- **Olive oil** if used while making tomato soup also helps absorb antioxidants.
- According to Johanna Brandit (In Grape cure), **Grapes** can cure cancer. The patient should be kept on light meals or on fast for 3 days and then grapes should be given not more than two kilos per day. Do not give any other thing to eat. After three days, normal light meals are to be given and buttermilk also should be given. Keep the patient on normal light diet for three days and again grape diet should be given for three days. This cycle of grape diet and normal diet should be continued for months to get good results. Some doctors suggest that for complete two months, the patient should be kept on grape diet.
- **Carrot** has been found to cure cancer. Its juice should be taken daily. It is good for stomach cancer and blood cancer. It has vitamin B, calcium, phosphorus and some sulphur. Regular use of carrot during its season purifies the blood.
- **Garlic** protects from cancer and also cures cancer, T.B., heart problems, influenza and polio. Two pieces of garlic should be grinded to a paste and mixed with water and then taken after meals every alternate day for at least 15 days. The results should be watched. A limited quantity of garlic mixed in the vegetables every day is beneficial.

- **Wheat grass** is one of the best remedies for prevention of growth of cancer growth prevention and for curing it. Not only cancer, wheat grass juice is beneficial for curing many incurable diseases. Dr. N. Wigmore, Naturopath of worldwide fame has written in his book that cancer is a state of body and it is not to be worried about. Wrong type of diet, wrong living, wrong atmosphere and wrong ideas bring in cancer. It can be cured by wheat grass juice. **To make this wheat grass at home**, wheat seed should be left in a number of earthen vessels to grow. Do not put any fertilizer in it and let it grow naturally. Within three or four days, grass of wheat would come up. Let it lengthen to 7 or 8 inches and then pull it with root. Cut the root and wash the grass clean before making a paste of it. Add water and filter it to make half a glass of this juice. It should be given to the patient empty stomach and then half glass of juice should be given in the evening. Do not give anything to eat up to two hours of taking this juice. The paste filtered out from the juice can also be taken with meals. Every time fresh juice should be prepared after plucking grass from the vessel. One has to keep at least ten vessels to grow grass of wheat. Every day one vessel should be planted with wheat seed so that every day you get grass from one vessel. Wheat grass juice is one of the best remedies for all urine problems, prostate cancer, kidney stones, blood pressure, cardiac problems, paralysis and skin problems.
- **Wheat grass** has now been made into a **homeopathic**

potential polycrest remedy and Dr. Sudershan Bhatti of Ludhiana has done a lot of research work on it besides curing many cases of various chronic diseases including cancer. In the preface of his book in 'Wheat Grass', he gives a case of cancer tumor in throat, which despite allopathic treatment, radiotherapy and chemotherapy did not respond. The patient was unable to eat because of spread of tumor and then was put on wheat grass medicine. It was a life-saving drug for the patient and she was cured of throat cancer. Dr. Bhatti has authenticated this case by giving address of the patient in his book so as to verify.

- Some scientists of National Dairy Organization have said that **curd** has properties of curing many types of cancer. Its daily use prevents growth of cancer.
- Those who have already found that cancer has attacked them should avoid fried food. Continued use of fried food and fully vegetables produce 'pyrogenic' agents that may cause cancer to those who are already prone to it.

VIEWS OF NATUROPATHS ON WHAT TO EAT AND WHAT NOT TO EAT

[It is advisable that a Naturopath should be consulted for proper guidance in diet.]

The research studies show that cancer is the end result of wrong eating habits and unhealthy living. This is on account of biochemical imbalance and physical or chemical irritation of the tissues. In our food, we have an abundance of carcinogenic substances. This added to deranged metabolism produces cancer.

If one checks the data of cancer of prostate, it is more in western countries where men consume animal proteins, particularly meat in their diet. Protein intake of more than 20 to 30 grams per day is not digested properly and acts as a poison producing carcinogen. As stated above, a complete overhaul of diet is very important for effective treatment of prostate cancer. Here is a specific list of food items to be taken as per views of Naturopaths.

WHAT TO EAT IN CANCER?

- Naturally grown foods which are free from carcinogenic elements should be taken. Foods containing man-made chemicals, toxic additives, insecticides and preservatives or artificial colors should not be taken.
- Sprouted seeds, nuts and grams, raw vegetables, soyabean, buckwheat millet rice and dried beans make a suitable diet for cancer patients.
- The best anti-cancer grams are millet, buckwheat, brown rice and barley.
- One can also take anti-cancer diet like fermented foods e.g. naturally fermented vegetables, fermented grains and also fermented juices.

- Some doctors also suggest that fifty to sixty percent of daily diet should consist of lactic acid fermented food.
- Easily digested proteins must be taken. These proteins are present in potatoes, sprouted seeds and grains, green vegetables, nuts and cottage cheese made from high quality unpasteurised milk.
- Raw goat milk of high quality contains anti-cancer properties.
- Processed vegetable oils like sunflower seed oil, flex seed oil and soya bean oil are useful. One of these oils should be added when food is cooked.
- Some vitamins should be added in daily diet. These are vitamin A, B_{12}, C and Potassium.

WHAT NOT TO EAT IN CANCER?

- Milk or milk products should be avoided except home-made cheese or soured milk.
- No animal proteins, meat, eggs or fish.
- No use of animal fat.
- The said oils should not be heated for long time when preparing vegetables.
- White flour and white sugar are refined carbohydrates. These should not be used for food preparations.
- Alcohol should be avoided.

NATURAL TREATMENT OF CANCER

- After evacuation in the morning, apply some mustard oil on your palms and rub both the palms together for about thirty times. This can be done two times in a day after evacuation in the morning and evening.
- Take 20 leaves of 'neem' (Azadirachta), 15 leaves of 'Bel' (Aegle marmelos) and 20 leaves of 'Tulsi' (Ocimum). Wash them all with water and grind them to express the juice. Take this juice with one tsp of honey each morning.

NANOTECHNOLOGY— A HOPE FOR CURING CANCER

Research in early cancer detection and treatment and its connection with obesity are recent findings by research scholars of US. According to the news item contained in Times of India, New Delhi, dated November 3, 2005, there is now hope that cancer can be detected in its early stage and that it can be cured as well.

Scientists are beginning to develop microscopic tools to discover and treat cancer. There are some general ways by which they hope to eventually use these innovations. The method is called **'Nanotechnology'.** Nanotechnology is the minutest element or curing agent encased in drugs that can be seen by microscope only. It is not a new term and NASA has used this technology in space journeys.

According to Nanotechnology, a sample of the patient's blood is passed across a device containing nanowires. The molecules associated with cancer will react with the nanowires signaling the presence of a particular type of cancer. The signal is relayed through electrodes to a computer and complete data indicating cancer is displayed on the computer. The early detection of cancer thus greatly improves the patient's prospects of survival. This procedure is for detection in the beginning of cancer.

GROWTH OF CANCER

Highlighting tiny clusters of cancer cells help doctors to detect whether cancer has spread or is shrinking in response to treatment, without the need for surgery. To accomplish this job, nanoparticles engineered to target cancer cells are injected into the body. The nanoparticles locate and then bind to the cancer cells. The particles, which are magnetic, allow the cancer to be readily detected by magnetic imaging or MRI. MRI allows doctors to see whether the cancer has spread to lymph nodes without surgically removing the lymph tissue. It could also be used to show whether treatment has cleared cancer from the lymph nodes.

CURING CANCER

Drugs encased in packages small enough to slip through cancer cell walls kill the tumor without damaging healthy cells, reducing the side effects of treatment. In the first instance, a nanoparticle containing a powerful anti-cancer drug is injected into the body. The particles are designed to attach to the cells of a specific cancer, while ignoring healthy cells. The nanoparticles attach to cancer cells and then release the anti-cancer drug inside. The anti-cancer drug kills only the cancer cells, while leaving the healthy cells undisturbed.

OBESITY AND CANCER

It is for the first time that obesity has been connected with cancer. In the US, roughly 10% of all cancers could be avoided if overweight and obesity did not exist, according to updated statistics on the proportion of cancer due to obesity. The new projections stem from a review of published studies and updates of the International Agency for Research of Cancer (IARC) report of 2002.

(All above data of Nanotechnology, courtesy news item in Times of India, Times International supplement of 3rd November, '05)

GENE THERAPY – ANOTHER HOPE TO CURE CANCER

Gene therapy is the latest invention in the field of medicines. It comprises of putting genes into the cells in the body, often to replace native genes that are malfunctioning. This therapy is already under field trials for the last fifteen years. The only difficulty faced by the innovator scientists is that they find difficulty of getting enough functioning genes into cells. M/s Introgen Therapeutics, an Austin, Texas biotechnology company has formulated a method in which tumor suppressor genes are put into cancerous cells to stop the growth of tumors. The company's most advanced drug, which is in the last stage clinical trials, is a treatment for head and neck cancer that it hopes will be the first gene therapy approved in the United States. In this type of treatment, viruses containing the desired gene are injected directly into tumors.

(**Courtesy:** *News item in Times of India, 7th Nov., '05*)

CHINA APPROVES NEW CANCER DRUG

Here is a news item from 'Times of India' dated 18th November, '05 which says, 'A cancer therapy using a virus that attack tumor cells but not healthy ones has been approved in China. The drug is essentially a copy of one developed and then abandoned by an American biotechnology company. A company of China, Shanghai Sunway Biotech, received clearance to sell the drug, *H 101,* in China as treatment for a type of head and neck cancer. H 101 uses a type of cold virus that has been genetically engineered to attack a particular defect of cancer cells. It is a modified version of Onyx-015, a medicine developed by a company of California.

NEW METHOD OF EARLY DIAGNOSIS OF CANCER AND DRUG

The doctors of National Cancer Institute of America have invented a new method to make an early diagnosis of cancer. Doctors may be able to detect cancer long before they produce any symptoms. This is by testing for the presence of certain gene mutation. Though, penetrating screening has led to earlier diagnosis in several cancers, current diagnostic methods are not perfect. A commonly used blood test for prostate cancer, the PSA test cannot distinguish between aggressive tumors and those that would remain slow growing for years leading to over treatment according to opinion of some doctors. A new tool called a **DNA micro array** allows scientists to analyze the pattern of gene activity in a cell. Using this information, scientists may distinguish between aggressive prostate cancers and those that are unlikely to cause any trouble.

A progressive advancement in imaging technique allow scientists to look at the molecular activity going on inside cancer cells, not just at their structure. Imaging, today, not only sees a lump, but a PET scan, for example, sees the biochemistry occurring within the tumor. Even its metabolism can be watched. Cancer cells use more of glucose than healthy cells. The PET scan, which creates an image based on cell uptake of glucose may be able to zero in on cancerous growth or detect angiogenesis within a tumor. PET scans can gauge whether a targeted therapy has shut off the metabolism of tumor cells. Now there is no wait for three months to know whether the patient is getting well or not because this method tells the doctor the condition within 48 hours.

Studies show that some men at high risk for developing prostate cancer may benefit from the breast cancer drug 'toremifene' or from taking green tea tablets. There are many more promising new cancer drugs available in USA, (Medicines like Gleevec, Herceptin, Tarceva, Velcade etc. for different types of cancer are awaiting approval for import in India) .

(Courtesy-article 'Winning the war on cancer' in Reader's Digest, Nov. 05 issue-concerned part on prostate only mentioned).

AYURVEDA AND CANCER TREATMENT

I happened to see an article on cancer treatment in Hindi 'Nirog Dham', a popular Ayurvedic magazine published in Indore. (Summer issue, 2005, article—'Hamara Ayurved Shastra'). The reference is on a seminar held on17th October 2004 on treatment of cancer. A medicine named **'Sarva-Pishti'** has been tried on many cancer patients with success. The medicine and research on cancer has been made by D.S. Research Center, 147A, Ravinder Puri Colony, Varanasi, India under the guidance and research of **Dr. Shiv Shankar Trivedi**. He has written a book named, 'Cancer harne laga hai' in Hindi in which he has listed those patients who have been completely cured by his medicine.

LAST WORDS ABOUT TREATMENT OF CANCER

We see patients of cancer dying all around us. If you visit cancer hospitals, you would find that the cancer patients are on the increase. We cannot do anything to save them. We see them turning into skeletons, getting bald and very weak day by day while under treatment. If you take the patient into confidence, in most of the cases, there would be some depression, some grief and some sort of mental ailment that has brought in cancer. Cancer patients have weak vitality and enfeebled nerve power. Every strain and worry lowers nerve power and makes the blood unhealthy. Taking nonvegetarian food, taking tea and coffee in excess, taking easy things to mind seriously (i.e. highly emotional), confining every problem in mind and not telling others the internal worries are steps that make easy entry of cancer in the body. If you want to take care of a cancer patient, be intimate with him or her to know the state of mind, console him or her and do not allow intoxicants including nonvegetarian food for the patient. Teach him to conduct 'Pranayam' and simple sitting exercises of 'Yoga' through a teacher and you will find fifty percent of patients responding.

■

SECTION - VI

PRECAUTIONS AND CARE FOR PROSTATE

Had breathing been an extra activity of the body without which one could survive, there would not have been time to spare for it due to busy schedule of people in big cities. It is not so and hence people have to breath in and out to live. This is a picture showing that we do not give much time to our health. This is one aspect and other aspect is that we do not respect our body. Suppose you are out to market for some urgent work and after a continuous exertion in Bank, LIC or other offices, you feel hungry and want to go to toilet also but you suddenly remember some work in IT office. Since it would be difficult for you to come again to this particular area you decide to do this work first and leave your urge to take food or go to toilet. This means that you have postponed your desire to eat and the impulse to urinate. This is one example. Now suppose you are on a bus journey and your water bottle is empty. You feel extremely thirsty. In the next terminal of halt for bus, you get down to take water.

There is no mineral water available in the shops but the municipal tap is running. You are afraid to take water from public tap for fear of taking contaminated water. You prefer to remain thirsty. Your body organs do not know why you are keeping them thirsty. This is another abuse of body.

But the greatest punishment and abuse to the body organs is when you prevent body urges and impulses. According to 'Unani' and 'Ayurvedic' therapies, following diseases occur when impulses listed below are stopped.

DO NOT STOP THESE URGES

When you stop	You may get major disorders or diseases like
Stool evacuation	Constipation, breathing trouble, pain in body, headache, gastric ailments, indigestion, eye diseases, eczema etc.
Urine	Renal calculi, prostate enlargement, pain in root of hair, Itching and eczema and all those diseases, which come after stopping stool.
Eructation	Hate to eat, trembling of body and hands, cough, hiccups
Sneezing	Heart sinking feeling, obstruction in neck movement, stiff neck, Bell's palsy.
Thirst	Deafness, dryness of mouth and lips,

	chest pain, tendency to doubt everyone, bodyache.
Hunger	Hates eating, body pains, tiredness and breathlessness on slight exertion. Loss of senses and change of skin color.
Cough	Asthma, anorexia, chest pain, nausea and hiccups.
Vomiting	All diseases of stomach, abdomen and skin.
Semen	Syphilis, eczema, psoriasis, depression.

POSTPONE THE URGE FOR URINATION AND INVITE PROSTATE TROUBLES

If you go on postponing urination due to your laziness or if you do not want to get up from sleep to urinate or if you hesitate to go for urination because of an important meeting or discussion in the office, you are developing a habit that is dangerous for your prostate health. Postponing the passing of urine puts pressure on the bladder and thickens its walls and then it leads to enlargement of the prostate gland. This also causes obstruction in the urethra. Many problems like total obstruction in passing the urine or interruption of urine (drop by drop discharge), burning of urine and pain while passing urine is common if the urge to urinate is postponed.

HAS TENSION ANY IMPACT ON THE PROSTATE?

Research indicates that we attract almost all the diseases through our inappropriate method of handling the tensions, which act like magnet for diseases. Under the tension regime in the body, there is release of harmful toxic chemicals stored in our body which cause fatigue, pain and disease. Tensions and worries send wrong signals to the body and the result is that we get increased frequency of urination or evacuation. Here is a practical proof. When a son is scheduled to return home by, say, five in the evening and does not return even after seven and there is no phone call from him, the mother gets worried with a psychological apprehension of tragedy. The result is that she gets frequent urination or evacuation. The same type of hormonal imbalance occurs in males and frequent urination is one great symptom whose impact on prostate can be harmful. It is very difficult to deal with tensions but once a man knows the way out, he gets free from diseases. The best way is to expose your problems to your friends, relatives or write them down to find out a solution. In response to tensions, we are uneducated. Repressing the tension and worry will not save us from body ailments. On the other hand, allowing in tension make us face external situations that confirm what we are experiencing. Avoiding the tensions, ignoring them, denying them or comparing them with the tensions of other persons as not the solution. This is just like a mouse who shuts his eyes and avoids running after it sees the cat. Tensions do bring ailments but they have a purpose to come. Tensions are meant to draw your attention to the unacceptable and your need to call for action. If you do so bravely and face the situation, tensions will not cause problems in your body. 'Difficulties are meant to rouse, not discourage', says William Ellery Channing, Psychologist.

DOES SEXUAL INTERCOURSE MAKE AN IMPACT ON PROSTATE GLAND?

Yes. During spells of experiencing prostatitis or knowing that your prostate is enlarged, better do not indulge in intercourse. There are some rules of this act. When you are not having any problem in the act of urination and you have not been to a doctor for check up of enlarged prostate and you are above the age of fifty five or sixty, you have every reason to enjoy sexual intercourse. Coition itself is an exercise for the prostate. It has to show its usefulness and get active. Any organ left unused for a long time is bound to get rotten. Prostate is no exception. If a man has not married, his life style is different and he has not used the sexual organs. In such case, prostate has negligible role. Married men with normal health can have sex but it should be during night so that a rest is obtained after this. There should be an interval of at least three hours after dinner otherwise gout, rheumatism, lumbago etc. can also aggravate, if existing. Do not have sex with a menstruating, pregnant or a diseased lady. Enjoy sex with wife only once in a month or so. **Those identified with enlargement of prostate should never go in for intercourse.** It should be clear that the prostate gland gives passage to the urethra and the two ejaculatory ducts. When the prostate gland has enlarged due to old age and its connective tissue has also increased, it may interfere with the emptying of the urinary bladder.

CHANGE YOUR LIFE STYLE

You have had a busy routine life and now are a retired person. Suddenly you have developed BHP and are now worried. You have spent sixty years of life in government service or in business and are not very active these days as you used to be in prime of your age. Your health is not very good but you must know that absolute health is not existing nowadays and it is because of polluted environmental influence, unhygienic mode of living, inherited ailments, drug abuses and ignorance of rules of maintaining good health on the part of people. It can be said that seventy to eighty percent of health depends on the correct mode of life-style that one leads. This will account for normal health if not absolute health. The rest twenty to thirty percent dependence can be made on treatment by medicines. Body is designed to conserve energy or its vital force provided its maintenance is correct. We have a system of security against diseases. Let this system be implemented. The health rules are: get up early in the morning, avoid late night sleeping, go for a walk in the morning, conduct some exercises, take balanced and nutritional diet and avoid excesses in every mode, be it food, sleep, sex, worry, tensions and so on. It has not been possible for most of us to adhere to these golden rules. **The word 'very' is troubling us at every step of life. We are 'very' busy, the life is 'very' speedy, the time is 'very' short and we want to get 'very' rich overnight.**

Having no time and being very busy, we opt for ready made food called 'fast food', tin-stuff and a variety of junk, smashing and storming the market. Our attitude towards simple but nutritional food has totally changed. We know we are eating bad stuff and still we cannot avoid it. We know that soft drinks are hard for our body system but still we go on consuming it. I cannot compel you to leave all this but can surely suggest some of the golden rules and attitudes which will keep you fit. The basic principle of healing in our ancient Indian books is that **one can create balance in the internal forces** working in an individual by altering diet and habits of living to counteract changes in external environment.

Our subject is prostate and we come to know about this when there is **indiscipline in urination.** The urinary system removes the water, salt and nitrogenous wastes of the body. It is formed in the large intestine and this waste product helps to maintain the normal concentration of electrolytes in the body fluids. The functioning of this system and output of urine depends upon our diet intake, water consumption, environmental temperature, mental state and physical condition.

VIEWS OF CONSTANTINE HERRING, MD ON URINARY TROUBLES

C. Hering was a great homeopath of his times in USA. In his book, 'Domestic Physician', he has given excellent hints about urinary troubles.

'It is strange to observe how anxious most people are about their having an evacuation from the bowels every day, without taking much notice of how often they pass water. Yet it is ten times more dangerous to go one day without urinating, than a whole week without a passage from the bowels. Never postpone the former business for any consideration whatever. Many people have died a very painful death from their having waited too long to urinate. It is astonishing how sensible people can run such a great risk on account of extreme modesty or bashfulness while attending church, parties, especially sleighing parties, concerts or other assemblies and when travelling. Do not be in a hurry when urinating, do not strain too hard, empty the bladder completely and avoid a cold draught. Consider that the few moments, which may be gained in this way, are out of all proportion to the time lost during a long illness, which may be caused by it. It is important to drink water often, particularly when the urine becomes more scanty. If the discharge of urine becomes for some time more and scanty, it is an indication of a disease, which may suddenly become dangerous; take everyday a warm foot-bath, drink plenty of water and now and then butter-milk; but beware of diuretics, such as gin, juniper berries etc. For constant desire to urinate, pain, burning etc., use application of warm water, a warm bath and mucilaginous drink, particularly oatmeal gruel and partake of nothing acrid, salty or sour.'

INCOMPETENT FOODS

In BHP, diet plays a vital role.

Diet should be selected according to individual constitution and the region to which one belongs. Food habits of South Indians and East Indians differ from West and North Indians. The basic food is rice and wheat. This need not be changed and should be according to the region where they live.

The best is to identify one's constitution and select the food. When thinking about diet, one should see that quality and freshness of food is maintained. Food should be taken in lukewarm condition and not cold. Cold food would bring more of urine.

- The basic principle of eating is 'Do not take food unless you feel hungry and do not drink water unless you feel thirsty'.
- 'Do not take food when you are thirsty and do not take water when you are hungry'.

There are some foods that are not to be mingled or taken together. For example, *fish and milk, meat and milk, sweet and salty, curd and beef, sour food or salty food with milk, sour fruit with milk; melons with water etc. are the combinations that are harmful for the body and bring in many diseases.* When these incompatible foods are taken together, toxins are produced and diseases like Leucoderma, Psoriasis, Tuberculosis and Cancer may result in.

SOME USEFUL SUGGESTIONS

- Get up from your bed as per your scheduled time. Do not jump out of the bed in a hurry. Sit on the bed with your feet touching the floor. Bring your hands before you, see your palms, rub them together twenty times and then sweep your face with palms upside down. Repeat this act thrice. Now thank your God that you had a nice sleep and that you are found living in this world after your death last night. Every morning God blesses you with a new life to start with, a new morning to resume your work. Sleep, you must agree, is like temporary death. So, take maximum benefit of this new day.

  (Purpose: By rubbing the palms and giving time to your body after sleep, actually you have given time to your heart to cope up with circulation activities ahead for the heart to exert. The heart was at rest during sleep).

- Drink at least two glasses of water without rinsing your mouth. It is better if the water kept for drinking in the morning is stored in a copper vessel the previous night. Switch on a radio or tape-recorder to listen to devotional songs in praise of your God. Walk around the room for a few minutes and go to toilet. (Purpose:

Preventing constipation, building self çonfidence and enhancing mental power).

- Prefer Indian style seat for evacuation. Defecate with ease without straining. During the act of evacuation, clutch your upper and lower teeth together keeping the mouth closed. This will strengthen the roots of your teeth. If you have a feeling that your bowel is not getting cleared, there are two methods, which your can try. Press the thumbs of both hands against the skin below the corners of lower lip. Continue pressure till you count twenty. Release the pressure and count ten. Repeat this act of pressing and releasing thrice. If this method does not work, try another. Put both hands on both feet so that the palms are pressing them. In this position, raise your buttocks upwards slowly to an extent that your calves and thighs make an angle of ninety or more. While raising the buttocks, take a deep breathing inside. Hold the breath for a while when your buttocks are in raised position and then release the breath out slowly as you lower down your hips. Repeat this act twice or thrice and you will have easy evacuation. *After every evacuation, you have to make effort to urinate. This is essential for the health of prostate.*

- Go for a walk. Do not walk fast. After this, return to your home and conduct 'Yoga' exercises as detailed in this book.

- Go for a bath. Warm water may be used in winters but immediately after the bath, avoid exposure to cold winds. In summers, try to take a bath in the open instead of a closed bathroom. Taking bath in the open has a freshness that is not obtained in closed bathroom. Dry your hair after washing to avoid sinus problem, if you already suffer from it.

- Before a bath, conduct the following activities: **Go for urination to empty your bladder.** Smear your right hand index finger with mustard oil and insert it in your umbilical opening ('Nabhi' in Hindi) two to three times so that 'Nabhi' is oiled. Now smear the little fingers of both your hands with oil and insert them in your ears so that the oil is applied on its inner walls. Do not pour oil in your ears. Similarly, with the help of right index finger, smear oil in both nostrils of the nose.

  With the help of left hand index finger, oil your anus, inside of it and the orifice. Wash your hands. Apply some oil on both thumbs of feet (first toes).

  (**Purpose:** Strengthening the intestines, preventing ears and nose from pollution-diseases, precaution against piles, **smoothening the bladder** by its emptying and other rectum diseases and taking care of eye sight by lubricating your feet thumbs).

- If you have a prayer place at home, devote two to five minutes in prayer and light 'dhoop' or 'agarbatti'. Pray to God for good health. You would get peace of mind.

- Your food and dress is the next thing. After breakfast, rinse your mouth with water five times so that all food particles are removed. Go for urination now. **Make it a habit to go for urination after breakfast, lunch and**

dinner. Rinse your mouth after lunch and dinner also. The best way is to keep the water in mouth and rub the teeth/gums with the help of your index finger. Using toothpick after a meal is a healthy habit.

- If you are a working man and your work involves lot of sitting on the chair, try to change your sitting posture every half an hour of continuous work or lean on the table. Slip to left, to right, forward and backward on the chair. Tilt and stretch your back and neck from time to time. Stretch your legs straight, move your neck sidewise, up, down and cover your eyes with your cupped palms for a while. If you are a retired man, you should not sit idle at home. Busy yourself by going for marketing of household goods, leaving and collecting children from bus stops, going to the nearest senior citizen club or library to read papers and chit-chat with your colleagues. If you keep sitting at home, this will **make your bladder idle and urine would stagnate**. Do not suppress or delay your urge for urination because you are busy in work or attending a meeting. **Never postpone the urge for urination**. Avoid letting the bladder full.
- At dinner, chew your food in such a way that it becomes a paste in your mouth and your intestines have an easy job to digest it. Do not watch TV and prefer not to talk much during dinner. After dinner, **go to toilet to empty your bladder (urination).** Return and sit erect on your calves, folding your legs beneath the hips and placing your palms on the thighs. Sit in this posture for fifteen minutes.

- If you are in the **habit of taking alcohol**, avoid it because it will irritate your bladder and may produce more of urine.
- Before going to bed, wash your face, hands and feet. Thank God that you had a good day. (Be it otherwise, always think positive). Do not cover your face with blanket or quilt in winter. Instead of this you can wear a cap, if required. Cold season may lead to retention of urine and increase the urge to urinate. It is **imporotant to stay warm** in bed in winters. Do not sleep on your belly.
- Eat whatever is your routine but make sure that you eat one 'Roti' or a little rice less than your desire to eat.
- Drink water half an hour before meals or half an hour after. If you cannot resist taking water during meals, you can have half a glass of water in mid of meals. Let me tell you an important point on drinking water. It is better if you **stop drinking much of water or beverages after 7-8 P.M**. Do not take tea or coffee after 6 P.M. Do not take any vegetable soup or vegetable curry. Even if 'Daal' is taken, make it dry and free of fluid.
- Try to make a habit of **clutching/pressing your upper and lower teeth together during the act of urination**.

When you adopt this type of life-style, you are going near to nature. If you are elderly, frail or have BHP, you do not need medication but need to build up vitality before being able to cope with this disease. Consult a professional. Let him decide to advice order laboratory tests for working of your system. **You should not worry about this disease because it is the doctor who has been hired to worry.** You have paid him for this job. Suppose he has advised that prostatectomy is essential but you can wait for some time since the symptoms have not turned violent after some medication. You can utilize the time between medication and operation of prostate. Change your life-style, go in for dietary changes, adopt nutritional supplements and improve upon your digestion according to your doctor's advice. You can take help of Allopathy, Homeopathy, Naturopathy and practice 'Yoga' as per your belief and confidence. In case, in this interval between medication and operation of prostate, the conditions improve, your doctor may tell you to postpone the operation. Believe it, this is possible with 'Yoga'and diet.

FIRST AID MUSCLE TONE TREATMENT FOR BHP

- In the early symptoms of prostate enlargement, one should do the following to tone the muscles of bladder and train it to empty itself. If it fails, think that the problem has to be given priority and doctor has to be consulted.
- Be relaxed during the act of urination. Better pass it while standing.
- When you feel that the urine has passed but still there is some more left in the bladder, keep standing and

wait for a minute or so. Try to empty the bladder again.

- Practice the above procedure of urinating waiting and then again urinating three or four times daily.
- Do it for seven days and if you find that bladder muscles have been toned, you are on your way to slight cure.
- If there is no relief, consult the doctor.

(Above References from Ruddock's Homeopathic 'Vade Mecum')

FIRST AID HOME TREATMENT FOR FIRST SYMPTOMS OF BHP

- In **retention of urine**, take four teaspoonful of **juice of Banana tree bark**, mix it with two teaspoonful of 'ghee' and give it to the patient. There will be immediate urination.
- **Retention of urine** can also be treated with **onions.** Take 50 grams of onions, cut them in pieces and boil them in one kilogram of water. When the water has reduced to half the quantity, filter the water through a cloth. A cup of this water mixed with one teaspoonful of honey, three times a day will bring the urine. Dribbling and increased frequency of urine are also cured by the use of onions.
- For **retention of urine**, take four pieces of onion and grind them to a paste. Mix the same quantity of wheat,

flour, as is the quantity of paste of four onions. Heat the paste of onions and flour for some time and then apply the paste on the abdomen while it is lukewarm.

- For **partial retention of urine** and frequent dribbling of urine when above juice is not available, eat a banana and then take half a cup of **Myrobalan** juice ('Amla' in Hindi) mixed with some sugar as per your taste. This juice is available in chemist shops of Ayurvedic medicines.
- In case your urine is **offensive smelling**, reduce your intake of salt immediately.
- In case of **scanty urine**, take 2 ounce of **Radish juice** twice daily besides increasing intake of water.
- Those suffering from **Dribbling of urine** should take **one Radish and one Turnip** daily in their 'salad'.
- In **Burning and retention of urine**,,half a glass of the paste like residue of rice (called 'Marh' in Hindi) while cooking should be mixed with some sugar and given to the patient.
- Take hot milk added with Jaggery ('Gurh' in Hindi) daily at bedtime. This will **clear the urine and treat retention.**
- For **retention of urine** and distension of bladder due to this retention, **Caraway** ('Jeera' in Hindi) and sugar may be grinded in equal quantity. One teaspoonful should be taken four times a day with cold water.
- There is a herbal medicine called **'Sheetal Chini'** in

Hindi. It is believed that chewing 4 to 8 granules of it and taking half kilo of water afterwards cures **burning of urine, retention of urine and swelling of prostate.**

(**Courtesy:** *'Nirog Sukh' Nov/Dec issue 2005, page 75)*

HYDROPATHY TO KEEP PROSTATE HEALTHY

You could even go in for Hydrotherapy, a part of Naturopathy for treatment of prostate. Hydropathy is a therapy wherein the treatment is with water, hot or cold.

Treatment of prostate is to have a bath in two containers (called sitz bath) having hot and cold water in each of the containers. The patient is told to sit in the tanks of hot and cold water by turn. One has to sit in the hot water tank and put his feet in the cold water tank for about three minutes and then sit in the reverse order for a minute i.e. sitting in cold water and putting feet in hot water.

Some naturopaths use cold and hot compress of a particular type of fabric or Turkish towel on lower abdomen and testes. Some naturopaths give stomach cleansing diet before undertaking this treatment. The purpose is to shrink the prostate and bring it to its natural condition. Cleansing diets help the body rid itself of waste products and environmental toxins.

Hydropathy should be done under the supervision of a Naturopath.

SELF EXAMINATION OF URINE TO KNOW THE CONDITION OF THE BODY

According to Ayurveda, the urine helps to maintain the balance of three humours, 'Vata-Pitta-Kapha'and water. Here is a clinical method to examine your urine for knowing the condition of your ailment, basically the urine affections and enlargement of prostate:

URINE COLOR TEST, VISUAL

- Collect your first urine early in the morning in a vessel. The collection should be mid stream. This means, the first and last stream is not to be collected.
- Yellow is the normal color of urine.
- Straw color urine is normal and indicates a low specific gravity under 1.010
- Amber color urine is normal and indicates concentrated urine with specific gravity of 1.010.
- Colorless urine is seen in large fluid intake, untreated diabetes mellitus, alcohol intake and diuretic therapy.
- Orange color urine is seen in concentrated urine, restricted fluid intake.
- Yellow foam may be due to biliverdin bile pigment.
- Red color of urine is due to hemoglobinuria.
- Brown black color is due to hemoglobin, Lysol poisoning or melanin.
- Smoky color may be due to red blood cells.

AYURVEDA INTERPRETATION

- If the color of urine is blackish brown, it is 'Vata' disorder.
- If the color of urine is dark yellow, it is 'Pitta' disorder.
- If the color of urine is cloudy, it is 'Kapha' disorder.
- In the case of BHP, the color of urine will be dark yellow.

SMELL TEST

- Normal urine has a particular uremic smell. If the smell is offensive and foul, this shows that toxins are present in the urine and the prostate is enlarged.
- The acidic smell of urine is an indication that you have urinary tract infection. Prostatitis is not ruled out here.
- If the urine is thick and has gravel, there is likelihood of renal stones.
- A sweet smell of urine and when you find lot of ants in the toilet seat, this shows diabetic patient.

OIL TEST

Now put one drop of sesame oil in the first urine.

- If the drop spreads immediately, the disorder is easy to cure.
- If the drop sinks to the middle of the urine sample, this means the illness is moderate but will take some time to cure.

- If the drop sinks up to the bottom of vessel, the illness is very difficult to cure.

SUMMARY - GOOD HEALTH OF PROSTATE

- Do not postpone urinating and evacuating for want of time. Do not suppress such urges and impulses. Avoid letting the bladder get full.
- Do not allow constipation to occur.
- Do not smoke or chew tobacco.
- When the bladder is full, do not conduct exercises, especially jumping and skipping.
- Do not have unprotected sexual intercourse if you indulge in sex act at in advanced age.
- Avoid sexual activities when having prostate problems.
- Eat foods that are rich in zinc, selenium, magnesium, vitamins 'C' and 'E'.
- Eat plenty of green vegetables and fruits.
- If you are a non-vegetarian, eat fish twice a week. It has fatty acids to boost immunity and gives protection against infections that is common in prostatitis.
- Eat enough beans and nuts rich in proteins.
- Avoid excessive fatigue, physical and psychological stress.

- No intake of tea and coffee especially after seven in the evening. It should not be more than two cups a day.
- Reduce intake of full cream milk, butter, ghee and refined carbohydrates.
- Must attempt urination before taking bath, after lunch and dinner.
- Conduct 'Yogasans' as detailed in this book.
- Do not take alcohol when prostate enlargement has been identified.
- Do not take excess of water after 6-7 P.M. and do not have a vegetable curry, vegetable soup or cold drinks before dinner. Any excessive water intake can increase urge and frequency of urine.
- People who are fond of taking milk while going to bed should stop this. They can take milk in the morning with breakfast.

■

SECTION - VII

YOGA AND PROSTATE GLAND

PRANAYAMA

The first sign of life in a newborn baby is to take a deep breath. This first breathing is called *Prana* because without it the baby cannot survive. This ritual is without any training to the baby who takes a breath inside, retains it for a while and then releases the breath. This is the process of breathing by which life commences. The life ends when this breathing ceases. One can live without food or water for sometime but one cannot live without breathing. To attain good health, breathing has to be controlled and vitalized by some method of breathing in and out. *Pranayama* is developed to look into this very aspect.

Our ancient books on health reveal that there are three steps in conducting Pranayama. Inhaling air into the lungs with all of one's strength is the first step called *Poorak;* Holding back air in the lungs is the second step called

Kumbhak; final exhaling of air from lungs is the third step called *Rechak.*

Poorak should be for about 10 seconds, Kumbhak should be for about 40 seconds and Rechak should be for 20 seconds. Actually this timing of holding the breath depends upon the capacity of the individual and is variable.

THE PRANAYAMA AND ASANS USEFUL FOR PROSTATE

Starting 'Yogasans' is very simple. Get up early in the morning and go for a walk. Return to your home, have a bath and sit for 'asans' on a mat in an airy room. Sit in either Sidhasan, Padmasan, Sukhasan or Vajraasan. You can learn these asans from some expert of Yoga. Padmasan and Sidhasan are explained below:

PADMASAN AND SIDHASAN

Spread a clean mat and sit on it. Fold your legs either in lotus asana (Padmasan) or Yoga mudra (Sidhasan). Lotus asana can be learnt from a person knowing Yoga. For this, you have to fold your left leg on your right thigh. Now fold your right leg over the thigh of left leg. Or you can do vice versa i.e. placing first right leg over the thighs and then the left leg over it. The heels will be beneath the navel region and the knees will be touching the earth. The soles of both the feet will be facing towards sky. Keep your back in a straight posture while sitting and spread your hands straight on your knees. Now fold the thumb and index finger of both the hands together so that the tips of both thumb and index finger touch each other. The rest three fingers of each hand will be resting on your knees. This asana is a little difficult but in due course of practice, it can be done with ease.

If this is found a little difficult, you can try yoga mudra. For attaining yoga mudra (**Sidhasan),** place your left heel beneath right the thigh so that the heel touches the middle area of anus and genitals. Mind it that this is the area of your prostate. Now, put your right leg over it in such a fashion that the sole of right foot faces the sky. Now, place your hands on your lap, on the heel of the right leg. The hands are to be kept one above the other facing the sky. Please note that the heels of the legs should not be kept over the pubic area. This is a much easier asana and can be a starter for doing your 'pranayama'.

PRANAYAMA

Pranayama is the process of breathing smoothly, inhaling and exhaling from the nostrils as per the following procedure

- Take a long breath slowly and exhale slow in the same way. Repeat it for five minutes. This is called **'Bharstika'** pranayam.
- Inhale through the right nostril and exhale through left nostril, using thumb and middle finger to close and open alternate nostrils by pressing side of the nose.

Do it for at least ten minutes. This is **'Anulome Vilom'** pranayam.

- Now comes the second step. Inhale through the left nostril and hold your breath for some seconds. Now release the breath from right nostril. For inhaling and exhaling from different nostrils, you have to use thumb and finger to close the nostril. Do not go beyond your capacity of holding the breath. This requires practice. The time for which you can hold your breath should depend on your capacity to do so and in no case should it be prolonged. This exercise creates a cooling effect in the body and increases the immunity. Do it three times only.
- Release the breathing out with slight force so that your abdomen goes inside with the intake of air and comes back in the same position during the next inhalation. This means you have to do 'Rechak' only. This is called **'Kapalbhati'** pranayam. Do this pranayam for five minutes. You can start for one minute and raise it slowly up to five minutes slowly after a few days.

SHAVASAN (CORPSE POSE)

[Shavasan is one of the best asana for relief in stress. Dr. Datey, a renowned heart specialist of Bombay and recipient of Dhanvantri award appreciates shavasan for releasing tensions. Explaining as to what happens when there is stress, he says," There is at once an impulsive reaction. Stress is communicated to the brain by the five senses. *Thalamus* further transmits the impulse through the autonomous nervous system. Impulses are modified through *Shavasa*n. The shavasan is the best form of relaxation; it even helps you to change your nervous system. You would not react to a crisis as an average person would. The shavasan was once tried on 47 patients with hypertension of various etiologies. A significant response was obtained in about 52 percent of the patients." (From the book 'Old age to youth through Yoga' by Dr. Siddhantalankar).]

Lie flat on your back on the floor and spread your feet keeping them at a distance of about two feet. Place a small pillow or folded blanket behind your head. Do not use a thick pillow. Your hands should be close to your body, touching the body. The palms should face upwards and hands should not be clenched. Close your eyes. Now feel relaxed and let your body be released or let loose. Try to feel the different parts of your body in contact with the floor.

For doing this, close your eyes and imagine that your entire body, part by part is in touch with the ground and is getting heavy. Do not get worried over this when you actually feel the limbs heavy. Throughout the practice of this asana, the worries and problems may keep appearing. Convince and tell yourself that these problems will receive your attention after a few minutes and that you are now practicing shavasana. Gently and slowly you will gain confidence and you will feel relaxed in all respects. During the asana, feel free and relaxed as if you are dead so far as your body is concerned. Remain in this 'shav' or corpse position for some time, say at least ten minutes without any movement. While you are acting like a corpse, breathe deeply and take long breaths.

YOGASAN FOR THE HEALTH OF PROSTATE GLAND

Prostate gland is located in such a place where it is difficult to make it mobile. Every organ has to be governed by contraction and relaxation to keep it healthy. It is essential for prostate to get flexibility, good circulation in blood vessels, arteries and muscles for its good health.

PROSTATE HEALTH ASAN I

It is possible to give some exercise to the prostate and the method is to conduct 'Sidhasan'. We have already explained this asan above. In it, the left foot is tightly pressed against the perineum and the heel of the right foot touches the pubic area. Perineum is the space between

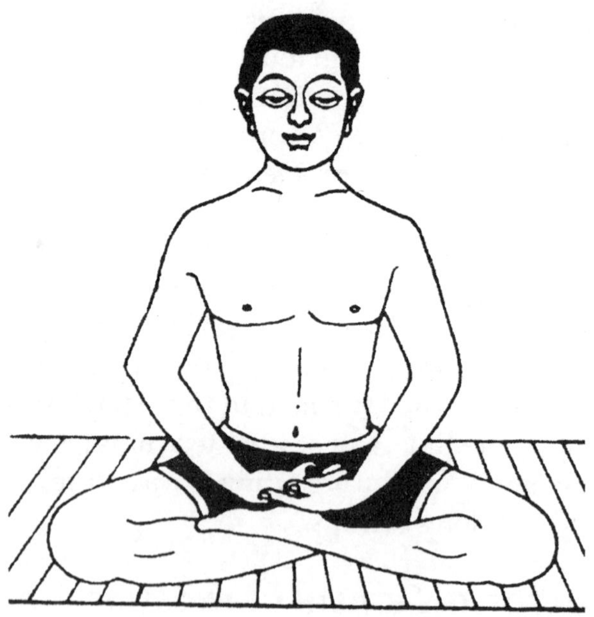

Fig. 6. Siddhasana — Sit with the left heel set against the perineum and the right heel on the left one

thighs, from anus to genitalia. This space is called 'seevan' in Hindi. When you conduct pranayam, you are sitting in Sidhasan for some time and practically putting pressure on the prostate. This is sufficient for the care of prostate gland since pressure for sometime would improve circulation of blood and keep it healthy.

One thing must be noted that 'Sidhasan' may not cure all diseases of prostate but it would prevent BPH and prostatitis.

PROSTATE HEALTH ASAN II

Place your chest on your thighs while pressing stomach with both your fists. Put you hand just above the pubic region above the penis. Now press the area and you would feel a bone. It is below the navel where the muscles of the abdomen end. It is here that the bladder is located.

Sit straight in erect position with your buttocks on your thighs. Your legs in this position are beneath the thighs. Now clench both fists and place them on your stomach around the navel. Breath out and bend down so that your chest is touching the thighs and head is near the ground. Remain in this position for a while till you can hold your breath in and then release the breathing and sit erect. Repeat this asan three times each day. This asan will exert pressure on the mouth of the bladder, which is surrounded by the prostate. Pressure from bladder side is a good exercise for prostate.

PROSTATE HEALTH ASAN III

Lie on your back on the floor and keep both arms on your sides. Now, raise your knees and move your feet closer. Place your feet together in such a way that the soles of feet join together. This will make your knees sink towards the floor on both left and right sides. With soles joined together, try to bring both the joined feet close to your buttocks, as close as you can do so comfortably. Hold in the same position for about three minutes. Do it every day. This exercise will stimulate circulation to the prostate and surrounding area. It is supposed to cure prostatitis as well.

PROSTATE HEALTH ASAN IV

Sitting on toes, joining both heels and sitting on the perineum.

Sit on both your toes in such a fashion that both heels are joined together and your toes are facing to the sides of your body and whole of the weight is on the heels. Now, you are sitting on your heels. The heels are touching the central region between anus and testes. This posture can be obtained only when you balance the body by holding some chair or table or wall with your hands. See that your folded knees are extended to both your sides. Now move your folded knees inside and outside while the heels are still on your buttocks. Do this 10 -15 times according to your capacity of balancing on heels.

PROSTATE HEALTH ASAN V

Joining both soles of feet while sitting and raising/ lowering folded knees.

If you have seen Swami Ramdev teaching various Asanas on your TV set, you must have watched him doing this asan during a recess time after you have done aggressive asanas. He has graded this asan as 'sookhsham' asanas and calls it the *butterfly asan.*

Sit straight on the floor and fold your knees. Now, bring your feet together and join them in such a way that the soles of each foot join together. Cup your feet at the dorsal end with both your hands as if you are cementing the soles together. Now pull the folded feet towards your pubic area as close as you can. Keeping this position intact with your hands pressing the feet, raise your knees above the floor and then bring them back to floor. Repeat this movement of raising and lowering the folded knees at least thirty times.

PROSTATE HEALTH ASAN VI (NYOLI)

Standing in bent position, placing both hands on knees and breathing in/out.

Nyoli is generally conducted for the health of stomach and abdomen because doing this asana stimulates intestines. This involves movement of abdominal muscles up and down and sidewise.

Stand erect and place both palms on the thighs by bending slightly. This posture will bring your body weight on the waist. Breath out and then contract the abdomen towards inside. Now, contract and relax your abdomen from above the pubic area by breathing in and breathing out. This would bring the abdominal muscles up and down. Do it for some time everyday. You have to learn it from a Yoga-teacher.

Note: All these Asana should be done in consultation with a Yoga teacher who should be told about your prostate problem.

■

SECTION - VIII

ACUPRESSURE AND PROSTATE

Prostate enlargement can be reduced and normal prostate can remain healthy if acupressure is done at the points of body wherefrom the flow of blood and veins join them to the prostate.

Our body has many vulnerable points, where the flow of blood counts. These points if pressed or punctured with the help of needles, normalize the flow of blood, if there is some obstruction in the flow or the flow is not regular. Basically it is thought that there has to be some obstruction in the flow of blood or the flow of blood is irregular in the body because of which diseases arise. In order to regulate the flow, some impact or pressure or puncture has to be made and for this, many therapeutical methods have been developed out of which pressure therapy is the simplest. Other therapies are *acupuncture, reflexology, shiatsu* etc. but the oldest one is said to be acupressure. According to a proverbial saying, acupressure therapy was initiated by saints of ancient India. It was developed here and then it spread to China, Egypt, Central Asia and other countries.

According to another belief, Buddhists had tremendous faith in this therapy and during the spread of Buddhism, they preached this therapy along with teachings of Buddhism in other countries.

Acupuncture therapy is supposed to be 5000 years old and it was initiated in China. In the ancient chinese literature there is mention of both acupressure and acupuncture and they claim that both the therapies originated from Chinese knowledge of medicine. Whatever may be the case, it is a fact that both the therapies are professed and practiced as a main line of treatment today in China.

You might have noticed that when a mother gets headache, she asks her children to press her head. This is the first –aid treatment in every home even today. It is also a fact that this application of pressure on aching limbs or head gives instant relief temporarily. This leaves no doubt about the wonder results of pressure by hands or by binding with cloth. Certainly, acupressure is born out of this pressure technique. Similarly, the birth of acupuncture has a different story. There used to be wars between countries during olden times where use of arrows and bows was common to fight the enemies. Leaving aside injury on account of arrows that used to heal if the arrow point was not on delicate organs, it was a surprising experience of soldiers to report that they were not only cured of their injuries but also of their old ailments of rheumatism, gout etc. This was a strange phenomenon for doctors to discover at that time and the result of research led them to acupuncture.

In the olden books of China, there are about 669 points of pressure listed for the treatment of various diseases but practical aspects of the therapy reveal 90 to 100 points of the body that carry more importance for cure of diseases. In twentieth century, this therapy was more or less forgotten. It was under the leadership of Mao Tse Tung in China that this therapy became popular.

Every tradition carried out from one family to another, from generation to generation has some sort of rationalism. Puncturing of ears and nose is a living tradition in Indian families. This is mostly done by women than men, who are not exempted. In Punjab and Rajasthan, men also get their ears punctured. These puncturing of ears and nose are not meant to wear ornaments and look beautiful. It has medical evidence that many ear, nose and heart diseases are averted due to this puncture. Many scholars of acupuncture therapy say that women are less prone to heart ailments because of this acupuncture. To avoid Asthma, even now people get their ears punctured. The result was that on ear itself, doctors discovered more than 200 acupuncture points. In 1950, a neurosurgeon, Dr. Paul Nozier developed exclusive ear puncture therapy, which is named as 'Oracular therapy'.

The scholars and doctors of India, China and Japan believe that life is a bioelectric phenomenon. This means that our life is based upon some life-electric-current or power. This power enables us to move, inhale, exhale, think and enact metabolism of body. Chinese call this power as 'Chi'. In India we call it 'Pran'. Homeopathy calls it 'Vital force'. This energy is of two types: 'Yin' and 'Yang'. Yin is negative and Yang is positive. With the help of these negative and positive balancing, the body remains healthy. In case of any imbalance between the two, the diseases occur. These negative and positive powers flow in the blood through a special route called 'Meridian'. Chinese doctors call this as 'zing'. There are 14 major zings in our body and out of these 14, twelve zings are in pairs and they are on the right and left sides of the body. The rest of the two zings are in the frontal central line of body and rear central line of body, vertically. Out of twelve zings, which are in pairs, six are Yin meridians and other six are yang meridians. Yin meridians start from fingers of feet or from the central part of the body and extend to fingers of hand and head. Yang meridians start from head, face or fingers of hands and extend to earth (feet). They also start from middle of the body and extend towards feet. In fact, this network of lines covers every part of body and as we press one place or point, the impact is transmitted to the organ which we want to cure. The only thing is that we should have adequate knowledge of points where actual application of pressure or puncture is to be made.

ACUPRESSURE IN TREATMENT OF PROSTATE ENLARGEMENT

There are seven points in our body upon which acupressure therapy is applicable and fruitful results have been noted. These points are as follows:

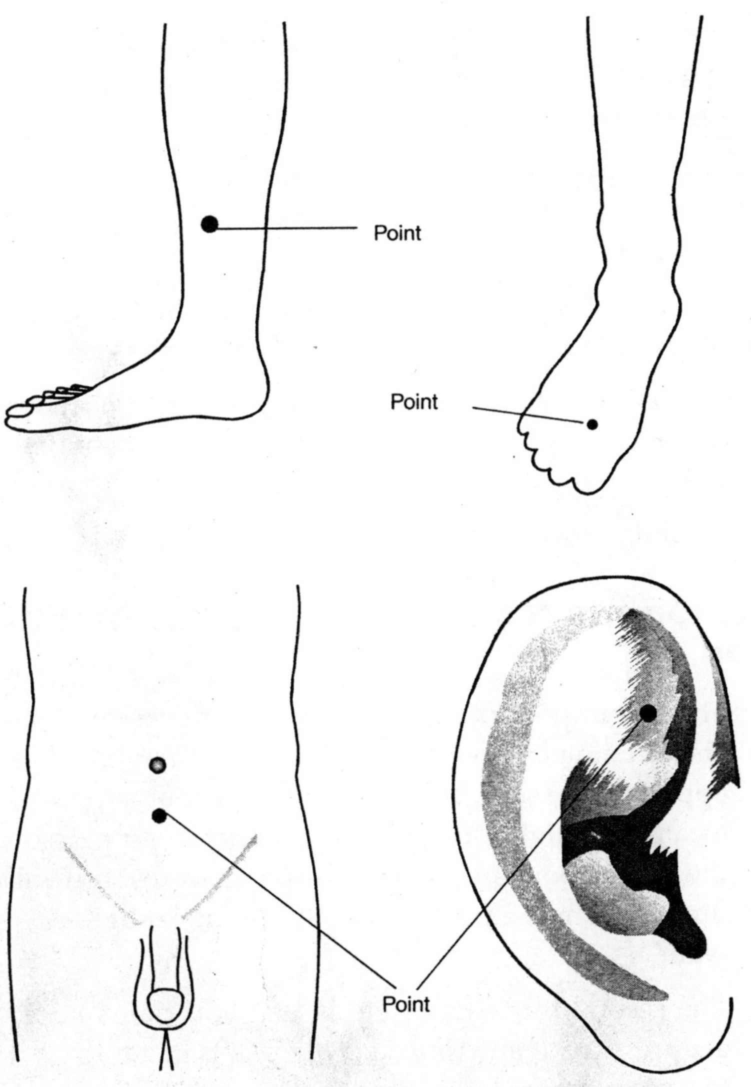

Fig. 7. Acupressure Points for Prostate Gland

- About two and a half inches above the ankle of feet (tarsal bone) on both the legs. There is one point each on the two legs.
- About two and a half inches above the area between first toe and second toe. There is one point each on the two feet.
- About three inches below the navel, just in the middle of lower abdomen, there is one point of pressure.
- One point each on the upper lobe of ears. It is above the opening of ear in the middle point of opening of hole and upper end-lobe of ear.

(Points shown in a sketch enclosed)

METHOD AND CONDITIONS OF PRESSURE APPLICATION

- The first important note is that if you have located the above points, there will be pain on the points while applying pressure. This pain indicates that the points located are right. In case you experience no pain on the located points, search for the point nearby. You will find one where a pressure would produce slight easy pain.
- The second important note is that you can conduct acupressure at any time and place. It is better to do it at a place where fresh air is available.
- The third important note is that you can press the point with any finger. It is better if pressure is made with the help of thumb, which can exert more pressure. If

you still want to utilize your index finger, better place it on the nail of middle finger and press the middle finger now on the point. For easy pressure, a sort of lever called Jimmy is available in the market, which can be purchased. Your nails should not be sharp or grown so that there is no scratch effected on the body.

- There are many methods of application of pressure. It depends upon the nature and extent of disease. The pressure can be applied by circulating the finger clock wise around the point or counter-clock wise or pressure from sides in an angle. But the most accepted and easy is **vertical pressure**.
- So far as prostate enlargement is concerned, it is better to apply the pressure vertically inside. The time for applying pressure should be for about ten seconds. Now release the pressure for 10 seconds and then again press the point for 10 seconds. Repeat this pressure and gap in between at least four times. Another easy method is to count up 13 slowly during the pressure period in your mind and release the pressure. Then again count 13 during the recess period before applying pressure again. The total time given for pressure should be 2 to 4 minutes at a go. This can be repeated two to three times in a day.
- In case the patient is tired and has come from outside work, is perspiring or his heart beat is more, allow time for rest before conducting acupressure.
- Immediately after meals, acupressure should not be conducted.

- If the patient has taken a hot or cold bath, wait for at least one hour.
- If the patient has come back from evacuation of bowels, it is advisable to wait for half an hour.
- If you have a fracture or an injured, acupressure should not be done on or near the place of injury.
- In case you have taken allopathic drugs, wait for two hours before conducting acupressure.

■

SECTION - IX

MAGNETOTHERAPY AND PROSTATE

INTRODUCTION

WHAT IS MAGNETOTHERAPY?

Treatment of ailments done by touching the magnets with the body for some time at particular ailing points is called Magnetotherapy. Magnet means attraction by means of physical touch. If the attraction is through mental power, it is **touch therapy** and if the attraction is through magnets, it is **Magnetotherapy**.

There is a flow of magnetic current in our earth. Modern science does not deny this. It is also well established by our ancestors that there is a link between the current of earth with the blood circulating in the veins and arteries of our body and that north pole of the earth has the power to control infections while the south pole of the earth has stored -energy. Keeping the current of the earth and the body in alignment, our olden mythological books (Vedas and Puranas) suggest that our head should be in the north direction while we sleep. Upon death of a person, his or her legs are drawn towards south and his/her body is placed on floor. These Hindu traditional rites are being followed since centuries and they have definite relation with earth's magnetic power. It is believed that death of a person is peaceful without much of pain if he or she is shifted from the cot to the good earth. This is meant to align the flow of the current of the earth in accordance with bioelectrical current of body.

Earth itself is a big magnet. If we suspend a magnet in the air, it will turn towards north-south direction due to the influence of earth's magnetic field. Earth has two magnetic poles: South and North. A unit called 'Gauss' measures the strength of magnets. In magnetotherapy, doctors use magnets up to 1500 gauss capacity. An instrument called gauss meter is available for measuring this. The magnet therapy has been valued and recognized by great philosophers like Aristotle and Plato. Even the father of Homeopathy, Dr. Hahnemann was influenced by this therapy. He used to carry a stick having magnets in his hand to examine his patients. Hahnemann was a man of letters who was in the habit of conducting various types of experiments to see that the patients get cured.

It is a known fact that during sleep, our brain and heart develop strong magnetic fields. Its strength is about 3000,000 kilogauss. This strength varies from time to time. Modern scientists utilize this magnetic field of the body for conducting EEG and ECG tests. The biological rhythm of heart and maintaining temperature of the body are partly done by the current of this magnetic field. When there is some disease, this magnetic field gets disturbed. According to magnetotherapy, blood (RBC) has about 4 percent of iron and when a magnet is applied on the point of disturbance, the magnetic flow in the blood changes and gets re-organized. This act of magnet application thus makes the body normal. When the flow of blood is normalized by this method, there is sufficient flow of oxygen and nutritional elements in the blood. The blood cells thus get strengthened. In some diseases of heart, lungs, kidneys and liver, increase of cholesterol, calcium and urea make the condition worse. With the help of magnets, these can be dissolved. Similarly, the diseases related with blood cells, pains, swellings, stiffness, bone pains and rheumatism etc. can be treated with the help of magnetic application. In the tissues of the body, there are ions. More of them are in the blood. These ions act as a good conductor of electricity. In the fat, bones and muscles the quantity of ions is less and they are not good conductors of electricity. This is the reason doctors of this therapy apply magnets on areas where blood, arteries and veins are more in our body. It is, therefore, essential for doctors to identify the potential areas where application of magnets can be made to full benefit.

RELATION BETWEEN MAGNETS AND BODY POINTS OF ACUPRESSURE OR ACUPUNCTURE

A magnet has two poles, positive and negative. North pole is positive and South pole is negative. There are many types of magnets available in the market. They are strong healing magnets, medium power magnets and curved low power ceramic magnets. Strong healing magnets are used for healing/curing paralysis, spondylosis, polio, lumbago, gout, sciatica and eczema etc.

About 14 mediums (meridians) have been selected in whole of the body as acupressure and acupuncture points, which we have already discussed in the previous chapter. These are divided into 12 couplets (paired meridians) and 2 singular meridians. Every point has a particular flow of magnetic field and when magnets are applied on these points, there is a positive response towards a cure. As a matter of fact, the acupuncture points are definitely related with magnet points in the body. Magnet therapy is called an allied science of acupressure/acupuncture because of similarity of points of meridians. Magnet therapy experts use these points as the areas of application of magnets.

In the acupressure, we have read about some points of body where pressure is applied. These are the points where magnet is to be used and besides these points, magnet is also to be used on soles of the feet.

USE OF MAGNETS TO CURE ENLARGEMENT OF PROSTATE

In the case of prostate disease, strong healing magnets are to be used.

- North pole is always used on the right side of the body and South pole is used on the left side of the body. Right sole is to be kept on North pole magnet and left

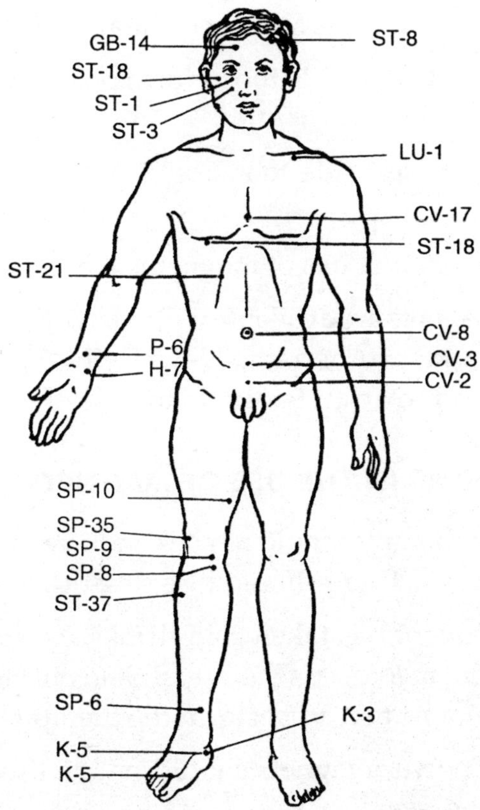

Fig. 8. Relevant Acupuncture Points on Front Side of the Body.

sole is to be kept on South pole magnet. The soles are to be kept on the respective poles of magnets while sitting on the chair. Ten minutes of use of magnets is sufficient in a day.

- The pressure point below the navel region in our acupressure detailing is called CV-2.
- The pressure point stated on leg above ankle is called SP –6.
- On CV-2 point, the South pole magnet is to be used.
- On SP-6 of right side foot, North pole magnet is to be used.
- On SP-6 of left side foot, South pole magnet is to be used.
- The duration of use of magnet is ten minutes.

The magnets are available with M/s B. Jain Publishers, Chuna Mandi, 10th street, New Delhi-55 along with guidance and relevant books on the use of magnets.

PRECAUTIONS IN THE USE OF MAGNETS

- Magnet therapy should not be conducted immediately after meals. There should be at least two hours gap.
- If the patient has taken cold drinks, ice cream or any thing that is cold, this therapy should not be done. Wait for an hour or so, to perform the therapy.
- Strong power magnets should not be used on brain, heart and eyes.

- Magnets of high power should not be kept together and should also be kept away from watches and clocks. Magnets should be kept in their containers.

Note: In the case of treatment of prostate enlargement, it is better to have guidance of a doctor of magnetotherapy. Without any practical guidance and demonstration, it is not wise to conduct this therapy.

■

SECTION - X

HOMEOPATHY AND PROSTATE

INTRODUCTION

The first question is why homeopathy? It is not that homeopathy is very popular and you have no other choice for any alternative system of medicine. It is not that the conventional system of medicine, allopathy, has totally turned you down. You have been advised to undergo operation and remove the prostate. Surgical operation on the body for any organ is recommended only when there is no alternative or cure. Removing enlarged prostate, hernia or appendix has become a need for the promoters of conventional system of medicine. We are told that we have no choice and this makes an impact on the patient. I have seen patients of hernia lingering on for ten years and more without going in for operation. In appendix cases, those who went in for homeopathic cure did not need any operation. If the case is of very urgent nature where infection has reached an emergency level, the operation has to be done. In the first reported cases of appendix, the cure by homeopathic medicines has been seen. In the case of BHP, homeopathy has helped thousands of patients forget about operations. One must not forget that we have an option before an operation is suggested. If the first symptoms in the disorders of urination are reported to homeopaths, there is no reason why an operation should be done in the later stage.

The main problem is our set up. We are trained to rush to allopathy for anything and this plugs a sort of confidence in the advice of doctors. If the doctor has advised operation, the impact is great. Psychologically, the patient has no choice but to follow what the doctor says. Even if you are not willing, your wife, son or daughter will make you undergo operation. You are the eldermost person in the family and head of family and still you are commanded by your kith and kin on this account.

Every disease has its onset, attack and decline or ends in fatal incident. Right from the onset of the disease like prostate enlargement, the patient gets enough warning and when the enlargement become so much that it obstructs the flow of urine, the patient goes to the doctor. He is told to get the prostate removed. You definitely have reasons to worry because your body is to bear the cuts, wounds and stitches for a number of days. Now a days such operations have become very easy and simple. But many people seek advice from alternative systems of medicines, perhaps with an idea that operation is ultimate and it has to be done but let there be a trial with alternative therapy. Why this thought comes to mind is simple to clarify. It is human tendency to avert surgery. It is in this zeal that homeopathy and ayurveda are put into grind. There are medicines in Ayurveda for curing BHP and I have seen people taking it. Not only in India, many USA drug companies advertise herbal medicines for curing enlargement of prostate. Herbs like saw palmetto or betasitosterol or Chinese medicines (He Shou Wu, Rehmannia from Yam tree etc.) are sold 'over the counter'(OTC) under different protected names. If you scan the Internet you would find many of the prostate medicines sold under guaranteed cure. I do not know whether these advertised medicines or Indian patent Ayurveda medicines containing herbs like Gokshura, Putikarnaja, Puga, Shatvari, Varuna and Akiki pishti etc. cure or not but I have knowledge about homeopathy in which people are using the medicines and have successfully averted the operation. In many cases, where the medication was taken in the early stage of enlargement, the shrinkage took place within four to six months and they have no problems. In advances stages, homeopathy has helped the patients avoid surgery by properly continuing the medicines.

One of the reasons to shift to homeopathy is one's inquisitive nature also. The second reason is that you want to see if better results can be achieved without repeating the medicines. You desire a permanent relief.

HISTORY OF HOMEOPATHY

Now you know the reasons why one shifts to Homeopathy. What is homeopathy? The oldest link and origin of homeopathy relates to the era of fifth century BC when a doctor called **Hippocrates, the father of medicine** invented two methods of healing, the *'contraries'* and the *'similars'*. There was a misconception those days that the ailments or illness was the punishment from the Gods. According to him, 'every disease has its own nature and arises from external causes, from cold, from the sun, from changing winds and that nature is the physician of our diseases'. His very theory that diseases can be cured by 'similars' was not accepted then and it remained in dormant stage for thousands of years. A German doctor, Paracelsus (1493-1541) went against the winds of his times. He saw the great earth as a chemical laboratory and identified the value of chemical experiments in medicines, both as the reason for understanding physiological processes and as a source of medicinal preparations. **Paracelsus was called the father of chemistry** because he desired to treat illness through pharmaceutical means. He based his study upon animals and minerals and rallied against those who believed that contraries cured. *He turned to German folk medicine, which believed in 'like curing like' or that the poison that causes a disease should become its cure."* In this process, he found that giving smallest dose of poison could cure the disease. This was not the law of cure in actual meaning, which was exposed by another doctor after more than two hundred years. It was Samuel

Hahnemann of Germany (1755-1843), **the father of Homeopathy** who made a history by change in treatment. He qualified as a doctor in 1791 and practised medicine for about nine years. He became disillusioned by the cruel and ineffective treatments of his time (blood-letting, purging, poisonous drugs with horrendous side effects). He had an inordinate thirst for knowledge and his greatest talent was for learning languages, mathematics, geometry and botany. In his routine work of translating, he came across translation of a book, 'Treatise on Materia Medica' by Dr. William Cullen. Cullen wrote about Cinchona's (a herb) ability to cure malaria. Following his 'like cure like' principle, he took this herb and experienced all the symptoms of malaria. This meant that cinchona produced in a healthy person the symptoms of malaria, the very disease that it was known to cure. This discovery paved a way for the homeopathic doctrine. During the next six years, Dr. Hahnemann conducted many provings on his family and friends and also studied accounts of symptoms by the victims of accidental poisonings. In his further practice he looked for the *similimum* - the remedy whose 'symptom picture' most matched that of his patients. His colleagues ridiculed him but he continued his efforts. It was unheard of in those days to give a single remedy when other conventional doctors made fortunes by mixing numerous substances, many of which were highly noxious. He used smaller and minimum doses for his patients. In 1810, he published his first edition of 'the Organon', which later ran into six editions. This book is supposed to be 'Gita' of Homeopathy.

Hahnemann was apparently a man of irritating nature and having an antagonism but in spite of this, he had many followers who had converted from allopathy to homeopathy. **Dr. Constantine Herring** (1800-80) was his first follower. He, who was told to write a paper disproving Hahnemann's theory but while studying 'Organon', he gave credit to the theory of medicine proved by Hahnemann. He was successfully treated by Homeopathy for inflammation of his hand that threatened amputation. He was thus totally convinced about Homeopathy. It was he who made a proving of a snake poison, Lachesis. After Herring, his next follower was **James Tyler Kent** (1849-1916) of America. His wife fell seriously ill and was treated by homeopathy successfully. He was a man with a high moral sense and remarkable energy for writing. Kent's books are dogmatic, like Hahnemann's later works. He advocated the use of very high potencies of medicines but like Hahnemann, his emphasis was on low potency like 30. He developed constitutional remedies and wrote many books of which his Materia Medica, Repertory and philosophy are even used today by all. Those doctors who use high potencies of medicines and follow Kent's methods of prescribing are known as Kentians. Homeopathy is now popular not only in USA, Britain but in Asia as well, right from India to Pakistan, Bangladesh to Nepal and SriLanka. It is now recognized as an official branch of medicine in India.

THEORY OF HOMEOPATHY FOR A LAYMAN

Health is a state of balance and disease is the result of weakness of the body's energy or vital force or the 'aatmik Shakti'. Once the vital force gets diminished, the body reflects the same in any of the diseases and one of them is thyroid disorder. The treatment is, therefore, aimed at strengthening the vital force so that the body itself heals the ailment. The symptoms of the disease are the main features for which the medicines are selected. The remedies are based upon the theme that substances produce some symptoms when they are given to a healthy person. When these substances in the form of remedy are given to the sick person, having the same symptoms, which a healthy person produced, the healing takes place. The principle is *'like cures like'* (law of similars). The remedies are made from herbs, plants, minerals, animals and other substances. The substances are repeatedly diluted, shaken or succussed by which the power of the substance is increased or one can say that the substances are potentized. *Potentization is the process by which invisible power of the substance is increased.* This sort of invisible power or energy stimulates the weak vital force because of the fact that it is of the same nature of which the patient suffers. It will nourish the vital force and restore the body to harmony.

SOME CONFUSION IN HOMEOPATHY

Those who come to the rescue of homeopathy have some confusion. Let us clear those confusions first to enable us to proceed further.

CONFUSION-I, IS IT SAFE?

Yes, it is very safe and free from side effects but let me clear that it is not safe if the doctor is inexperienced. Please note that Kent, of whom we have already read, said that he would rather share a room with a nest of vipers than be subjected to the administration of medicine by an inexperienced homeopath.

If someone takes a wrong medicine over a period of time, there is possibility of proving the medicine, which means some reaction. He will suffer from the symptoms, the medicine is supposed to induce and the cure will not ensue.

It is not safe if the patient does the medication by himself, after knowing the name of the medicine prescribed by the doctor. Overuse of a remedy is also not safe.

CONFUSION-II, IS IT SUPPRESSION?

Homeopathic medicines do not cause suppression. Suppression is uncommon in homeopathy but is possible if the doctor does not give oral medicines and directly goes in for local applicants or allows allopathic creams (cortisone for example) in skin diseases. Allowing application of allopathic ointments and giving homeopathic medicines internally may eliminate the skin disease temporarily but the disease will return. Poor choice of remedy also leads to suppression.

CONFUSION-III, IS IT THE PLACEBO EFFECT?

Some people say that homeopathic remedies have the placebo effect. A placebo is a pill without medicine. If you want to check its potential, give it to a person having non-bleeding head injury or in earache/toothache. The pill would not relieve the pains. Only a correcting selected remedy would work in these cases. Homeopaths utilize the placebo when high potency dose is administered to the patient and repetition is not desired. In between the interval of high dose and the time of next induction, placebo is used so that the patient is satisfied that he or she is taking medicine continuously. Noble homeopaths do not use placebo and tell the patients directly to come after a month or so for the next medicinal dose. In today's commercial era, this is not being done.

SUGGESTIONS ABOUT HOMEOPATHIC MEDICINES

If you are not a doctor and want to start medicine for enlargement of prostate, I would suggest you to start taking **Sabal Serrulata mother tincture**, eight drops in 1/4th cup of water three times a day. Take the medicine half an hour after breakfast, lunch and dinner and do not take anything for fifteen minutes after taking the medicine. Continue the medicine for 10 days and then go to the doctor for further treatment. You will surely have some relief.

Following is the list of medicines that are useful for enlarged prostate, prostatitis and allied urine problems. These medicines should be taken under the guidance of a doctor.

1. SABAL SERRULATA, MOTHER TINCTURE

This is the **prime medicine** for prostatic troubles. This medicine is to be taken in a dose of 8 drops in 1/4th cup of water, three times a day after half an hour of breakfast, lunch and dinner. After fifteen days, it can be reduced to two times a day on the advice of the doctor. At the onset of disease, it is very useful for enlargement or swelling of prostate gland. It has been found very effective in prostatic troubles in old age. The main symptoms of this remedy are enlargement of prostate, discharge of prostatic fluid, atrophy of testes, loss of sexual power, dysuria, enuresis, constant desire to pass urine at night, cystitis with prostatic hypertrophy.

There are patients who are taking this medicine for the last three years and do not have any prostatic troubles. There are no side effects reported.

2. THLASPI BURSA MOTHER TINCTURE

This medicine can also be given in the same fashion

as detailed in Sabal above. Like Sabal Serrulata, it is a specific medicine for urinary troubles. The main symptoms are frequent desire to urinate, heavy phosphatic, chronic cystitis, dysuria, spasmodic retention of urine, hematuria, renal colic, urethritis, urine runs away in little jets. This remedy, when used under the advice of a doctor **often replaces the use of catheter.**

3. FERRUM PICRICUM 3X

It is also a very effective medicine for old men with enlargement of prostate. The symptoms are frequent micturition at night with full feeling and pressure in the rectum, smarting at the neck of the bladder and penis, retention of urine and pain along the entire length of urethra or urethritis.

This medicine is not in liquid but in powder or tablet form. The dosage given on the bottle of the medicine should be taken i.e. thrice daily in acute cases and two times a day as preventive maintenance dose as per advice of the doctor.

4. PAREIRA BRAVA MOTHER TINCTURE

This medicine has also been used with good results for enlargement of prostate. The main symptoms of the medicine are black, bloody and thick urine, constant urging, great straining, pain down the thighs while making the effort to urinate. The patient can emit urine only when he goes on his knees, pressing the head firmly against the floor; bladder feels distended and dribbling continues after urination with violent pain in glans penis.

5. CANTHARIS 30

This is not a specific medicine for enlargement of prostate but it is an excellent remedy for prostatitis and associated problems of prostate. The symptoms are: intolerable constant urging to urinate, dysuria, bloody urine passing in drops, pains before, during and after urine; urine scalds and is passed drop by drop. In acute cases, four pills to be taken three times a day and then reduced to two times a day. The advice of doctor in the above symptoms should be taken after one day of taking the medicine because the symptoms of this medicine are not those of enlargement that can wait but these are associated symptoms that can become chronic if ignored. In Urinary Tract Infection (U.T.I.), this is one of the best first-aid remedy.

6. PRUNUS SPINOSA 3X

This medicine is quite useful in prostatic troubles. The main characteristics of the medicine are that urine appears to reach as far as glans and then returns. The patient has to force for a long time before it appears. The patient must hurry to urinate.

This medicine is in powder or tablet form and should be taken as has been described in the case of Ferrum Picricum.

7. THUJA

This medicine has a good reputation with prostate problems. The main action of Thuja is on skin and genito-urinary organs. When the urethra is felt swollen; prostatitis or urethritis exist; urine flow is scanty and it splits also, there is sensation of trickling of urine after micturition; severe cutting pain after urination, frequent urination with pains, desire for urine is sudden and urgent but cannot be controlled, under such conditions Thuja is useful.

8. CONIUM MACULATUM

Conium has a special affinity for old persons who have experienced sudden loss of strength while walking and painful stiffness of legs etc. Such condition is often found in old age when weak memory, sexual debility, hypochondriasis and urine problems are found. There is dribbling in old men, difficulty in voiding urine, urine flows and stops again; the discharge is interrupted and there is great debility in the morning in bed. The remedy acts on the glandular system, engorging and indurating it, altering its structure like scrofulous and cancerous conditions. It controls enlarged glands. Conium is a wonderful remedy if other symptoms of the patient also correspond.

9. STAPHYSAGRIA

Like Thuja, this medicine is useful in diseases of the genito-urinary tract and skin. Those who are very sensitive and have a history of sexual sins and excess fall within the purview of this remedy. The symptoms are cystitis, ineffectual urging to urinate when the bladder seems full, sensation as if a drop of urine was continuously rolling along the channel, burning in urethra during micturition; prostatic problems, frequent micturition, burning in urethra when not micturating (urethritis) and urging and pain after micturating.

10. CHIMAPHILA UMBELLATA

The medicine acts principally on genito-urinary tract and kidneys. When the urine is scanty, loaded with ropy, muco-purulent sediments and prostate gland is enlarged, this medicine is useful. Other symptoms are: urging to micturate, urine turbid, offensive, burning and scalding during micturition and straining afterwards. The patient must strain before the flow of urine starts. Acute prostatitis, retention and sensation of ball in the perineum are the other symptoms. The patient cannot urinate without standing with feet wide apart and body inclined forward. General use of this medicine is for loss of prostatic fluid, irritation of bladder and prostatic enlargement.

There are many other medicines like **Aloes, Alumina, Selenium, Benzoic acid, Natrium carb., Mercurius dulcis,** etc. and the same are to be taken according to their symptoms under the guidance of a doctor.

By use of homeopathic medicines, you can cure enlargement of prostate, prostatitis, related problems of urine, urine tract infection, calculi of prostate, painful urination or hematuria within a considerable time period.

In the case of enlargement of prostate, the patient can have a sonography before and after the treatment so as to ascertain the decrease in size and weight of prostate. Even if the size of prostate or weight of the prostate is not altered, the main benefit of use of homeopathic medicine will be that the patient would not feel any problem in his urination. When this happens, think that the size and weight of prostate is either returning to normal or it has lost its effect over the urethra making the urine flow freely. Forget about surgical removal of prostate at this stage.

VIEWS OF SCHOLARS AND AUTHORS OF BOOKS OF HOMEOPATHY ON MEDICINES FOR PROSTATITIS AND BHP.

1. Clarke

Enlargement: *Cann-i., Chim., Sabal., Solid.*

Senile enlargement: *Arg-met., Arg-n., Ferr-pic.*

2. Boenninghausen

Prostate affections: *Acon., Aspar., Bar-c., Caps., Chin., Clem., Cub., Dig., Nat-s., Puls., Rhus-a., Thuj.*

3. Pierce

Enlargement and inflammation: *Chim., Con., Cub., Dig., Lyc., Puls., Staph., Thuj.*

4. Boericke

Enlargement: *Ferr-pic.* and *Thuj.*

Prostatitis: *Merc., Pic-ac., Sabal., Staph., Thuj.*

5. R.B.Bishambar Das

Prostate enlargment: *Acon., Arn., Bar-c., Bell., Cann-i., Con., Dig., Oci., Pareir., Phos., Sabal., Solid., Spong., Staph., Thuj.*

6. Chatterjee TP

BHP: *Bar-c., Calc., Chin., Con., Dig., Hydrang, Puls., Sabal.*

7. Shinghal J.N.

Prostatitis: *Chim., Con., Ferr-pic., Sabal., Thuj.*

BHP: *Bar-c.*

8. Bhattacharya

BHP: *Ferr- Pic. 3x, Pic-ac.* 3x

Prostatitis: *Chim-Q., Merc., Nit-ac, Puls., Sabal, Thuj.*

9. Ghosh N.C.

BHP: *Arg-n., Aur-m-n., Bar-c., Chim., Con., Merc., Thuj.*

Specific: *Sabal.*

Senile: *Ferr-pic.*

10. Kent

Senile BHP: *Aloe, Bar-c., Benz-ac., Con., Dig., Iod., Nux-v., Sabal., Sel., Staph., Sulph.*

BHP: Fifty-one general medicines and hence not mentioned.

11. Dewey

BHP: *Sabal.*

12. Khokhar

Senile BHP: *Pic-ac.* 3x or *Ferr-pic.* 3x

13. Anshutz

BHP and Prostatits: *Hydrang.* Q, *Pic-ac.* 30, *Calc-f.* 6x, *Polytr.* Q.

14. Nash

BHP and Prostatitis: *Benz.-ac, Chim., Staph,*

CONCLUSION ON IMPORTANT REMEDIES AS SUGGESTED BY THE ABOVE AUTHORS

The above mentioned authors and scholars of homeopathy have graded the medicine for treatment of prostate enlargement. These are fourteen of them and marks have been given to each remedy excluding those which have **less than 4 marks.** No consideration has been given separately for BHP and prostatitis and both the diseases have been united to make a count. It is a joint calculation for both BHP and prostatitis

Marks for each remedy

Staph.: 4/14,

Ferr-pic.: 5/14,

Chim.: 6/14,

Thuj.: 7/14,

Bar-c.: 6/14,

Pic-ac.: 4/14,

Con.: 6/14,

Dig.: 4/14,

Merc.: 3/14,

Puls.: 4/14,

Sabal.: 9/14.

Sabal serr. for BHP– Marks : 9/14

Thuja for both BHP and Prostatitis — Marks 7/14

Thus, Sabal serrulata and Thuja appear to be the best two remedies out of fourteen for BHP and prostatitis.

■

MISCELLANEOUS

FORGET ABOUT PROSTATE PROBLEMS AND OLD AGE

If you are above fifty years of age, follow the routine as suggested below:

- Keep yourself busy even after retirement. Continue to inculcate new hobbies, new areas of living (change of station at times) and try to be in company of someone, your friend, your colleague in the office to avoid loneliness.
- Feel young. It is not the body that gives birth to thoughts but thoughts make the body. Be determined that you will live long and you will. You have tremendous divine power in your conscious. Utilize this power and have faith in God. Inhale fresh air and bask in the early sun light of the morning. Do whatever exercise you like to give enough contraction and relaxation to your body muscles.

- Leave all addictions. Leave smoking and drinking or chewing tobacco. Drink lot of water and eat balanced food. Take vitamin B complex and vitamin A tablets regularly under the advice of doctor besides taking nutritious food.
- Eat less and eat on time. Chew the food properly and clean the teeth with toothpick after every meal. Avoid too much of salt and sweets.
- Be a strict vegetarian. Take curd and milk everyday and keep the bowels clear. Observe a meal fast every week and eat plenty of fruits on the fast day.
- Observe celibacy after the age of fifty.
- Speak the truth to avoid tension of lies.
- Do not get involved in affairs of others and keep a distance from police and courts. Do not interfere in the matters of children and younger generation. No advice should be given to anyone till sought from you.
- Do not walk fast. Forget about hurry and worry. Avoid entering crowded places without company and observe fix timing for morning and evening walk.
- Consult the doctor immediately when not feeling well.

Last words

WHO ARE MORE PRONE TO PROSTATE PROBLEMS?

'Nothing is less worthy of honor than an old man who has no other evidence of having lived long except his age', says Seneca.

During my homeopathic practice in different states of India and abroad, I have observed varied attitudes of silver haired old persons. It was wonderful to meet them and get their experienced talks loaded with the woe of ailments when I was young. When I got old, it was still exciting to note their attitudes and share their joys and sorrows being in the same category of retired life. Senility has varied moods like glory and grief, joys and sorrows, maturity and innocence, childlike and childish, relaxed and obstinate. Old persons develop their habits, mostly disciplined, during the years of their blooming from teens to sixties. The span of nearly forty years between teens and sixties make them matured in every aspect of life but when they come to doctors, they behave differently. I have made serious observations regarding my patients and would like to share them with you.

(a) Some persons are very humble but look very worried. They come alone and tell their kith and kin not to accompany them to the doctor. They greet the doctor with folded hands and take permission to sit on the chair before relating their health condition. Their first request is to provide them an instant recovery even if it was a simple cold. They know that a common cold would be cured within three days of its own but still they wish it is gone within a day. They are naturally very sensitive regarding their healthy and on small disorders, they will rush to the doctor. They are harmless, simple minded and the advantage for them is that they do not get unwell soon. But when they get unwell, they create hell of the disease. Such type of people **do not suffer from chronic diseases or BPH and the reason is their full attention to the disease at the onset.**

(b) Some persons will only come with their sons/daughters or grandchildren. Even if they were seriously ill, they would postpone their visit to the doctor till their relatives accompany them. They are shy of telling their problems and would like to have a say through their relatives. Once their illness is told, they keep silent and simply make nods in affirmative or otherwise. The beauty of such gentlemen is that they keep smiling and listening. Others love them like adults love children. **They also do not fall sick soon and are not prone to BPH.**

(c) Some other persons are also hesitant to come alone because they cannot walk and hiring a rickshaw or auto does not suit their attitude. They are misers and would not like to spend a single rupee. Coming alone to the doctor means spending money, which they would not. They talk more about the discomforts of domestic life than their ailments. They need a listening ear rather than medical attention. They have not adjusted to life at home after retirement. What they need is company and not medicines. They are talkative and one must listen to them before they listen to you. I have treated many such persons initially with a dose of medicine for constipation, which is common in all senile problems. Later on, all their problems subside. They like to be examined physically, by stethoscope, pulse examination, measuring of blood pressure, etc. They declare you a very good doctor if you do that. They are misers but open-minded and expel their woes by talking. **They are not prone to BHP.**

(d) Some persons have general senile problems like anorexia and insomnia. They have a notion that they are not eating what they used to when they were employed and not retired. According to them, their appetite should be the same. This is the type of anorexia, they complain of. They sleep well in the afternoon and thus compensate their night sleep but still complain of insomnia. Such patients are living in the past. They do not want to face retirement and want to live in their pre-retirement era. Such people need consolation. Their need is good food and not much of food, good sleep and not much of sleep. Prescribing biochemic 'Five Phos' or 'Alfalfa' is what they need. These medicines should be given under patent labels so that they can read that they are being given tonics. **Such persons are not prone to BHP.**

e) Some persons come alone on their bike or bicycle. They are well dressed and have colored their hair to show that they are young. They wear light colored spectacles and deep colored clothes or jeans to show that they are still young. They speak nicely, greet the doctor and use gentle words of respect for the doctor. In due course of talks, they casually tell about their poor sexual performance. Actually they suffer from an illusion that they are still young. In the same category there are other persons who complain of spermatorrhea or involuntary emissions. In both the cases, they suffer from 'self-abuse'. They dwell upon sex, pornographic literature or films. They are weak in memory, have constipation, indigestion and have sunken eyes with loss of shine in their faces. The strange thing is that they do not reveal any other complaint other than the sexual performance or involuntary emissions. I have met such persons in the age group of seventy years and above. In most of such persons, the urinary problems exist and they suffer from BHP. **This is the category of persons who are very much prone to BHP and other urinary problems.**

I do not say that the persons belonging to 'e' category are the only ones prone to BHP. Persons from 'a' to 'd' can also have BHP. What matters more is the degree of the disease. **Every category can have BHP but those concerned more with sexual sphere even after retirement fall an easy prey to BHP.**

❖❖❖

BIBLIOGRAPHY

Organon of medicineand Chronic diseases, S. Hahnemann.

Lectures and Repertory, J.T. Kent

Boenninghausen's therapeutic pocket book, H.A. Roberts and Annie C. Wilson

Book of Surgery, Baily and Love

Atlas of Anatomy, Trevor Weston

Operative surgery, S. Das

Human Anatomy, David and others

Pathology, Virginia A. Livoci and others

Comparative Materia Medica and Therapeutics, N.C. Ghosh

Plain talks on Materia Medica with Comparisons, Willard Ide Pierce

Homeopathic Materia Medica and Repertory, W. Boerick

Prescriber, John H. Clarke

Materia Medica, C. Herring

Select Rour Remedy, R.B. Bishamber Das

Bedside Prescriber, J.N. Shinghal

From Old Age to Youth Through Yoga, S. Siddhantalankar

The Principle and Art of Cure by Homeopathy, H.A.Roberts

Science of Homeopathy, George Vithoulkas

Highlights of Homeopathic Practicing, T.P. Chatterjee

Chumbuk Chikitsa, M.T. Santwani

Ayurveda, Science of Self-healing, V. Lad

Acupressure, Dha. Ra. Gala, D.Gala and S. Gala

Wheat Grass, Sudershan Bhatti

Cancer, Causes, Treatment and Cure, Sultan Alam M. Bihari

Cure of Tumours by Medicines, John H. Clarke

Oral Diseases, Shiv Dua

Neck Pain, Cervical Spondylosis, Shiv Dua